MW01231006

Fight Through It

By Jared Weiss

The story of my life and how I overcame a life-threatening illness, my path to healing, as well as what I have learned throughout my journey-- most notably that nothing worth having comes easy and that there is divine meaning and purpose in everything.

Table of Contents

Jared Weiss

Goals for Sharing My Story

As you read my story I feel that it's important to tell you my hopes for sharing. I hope that you can use this for strength when times get tough...remember to keep fighting and to never give up. Never give up on your dreams, never give up on your loved ones, and most importantly never give up on yourself and your life. We all have a purpose in this world and I know that at times our visions can get clouded and it seems impossible to see it, but we have to keep moving forward and understand that setbacks can serve as the springboards for our major comebacks. I know that for me, whether consciously or unconsciously, whenever I experience a difficult situation or I am embarking on a challenge, I think, "Are there comparable situations that others have gone through?" (even though every situation and every individual is different). Or "Is there a quote out there or someone's words that can help get me through this?" I want this story to serve as your inspiration. Anything is possible and I am proof. When the doctors say you might not make it, and then when you do, that you might never recover completely—when others tell you that your dreams are too big, when others tell you that you are too small to achieve athletic feats, and when the world provides you with seemingly insurmountable circumstances to keep living—remember me and my story. When the world tells you to give up, refer to this. And when you don't think you can keep going, remember that your story is not over until you win!

The Need to Express Myself

A lot of what I went through during the most challenging times was unseen by others. It was beneath the surface. So when I would tell people who didn't know me about how I was healing from health issues, they would look at me and say, "Well, you look great." But that wasn't the whole story. You never really know what someone is going through just based on the outside. Also, when these difficult times leave us scarred, these scars can be visible or invisible. Nevertheless, they remain in our brains and subconsciously become part of who we are. We will always remember what happened to us and what we had to get through to achieve our success. The unseen can be just as, if not more painful and difficult. Be understanding of all, and realize that you may never know what someone is really going through inside, but we can always be kind and help others when it is needed.

I love getting feedback and people telling me that my experiences, videos, or my writing helped them get through their own challenges, or that it helped them get started on their goals, or even just that it injected some positivity into their day. If I did any of that in this book, then I feel I did my job. And oftentimes I'll look back on my words and peoples' comments on a post of mine, or old text messages when I need a spark to get back up when I'm feeling down. My words hold me accountable. In times when I don't feel good I remember what I tell others, and that gets me through. I hope to always be a positive influence in the lives of others!

SNEAK PREVIEW OF WHAT'S TO COME
Chapter 1

I think the only right way to tell the story of my life is to give you a sneak peak of the most life changing event in it. Let's start with a bit of backstory…in August of 2014 I was on my way to Cornell University after a grueling senior year of high school followed by one of the most amazing summers of my life. At the camp where I worked, I met the people who would later on become my best friends. We shared so many amazing times, and everything just went so perfectly. I said my goodbyes to the incredible summer and took the long car ride up to Ithaca where I was ready to embark on a new journey into college life. Shortly after arriving, I made my way around campus, first visiting the gym and getting into some pickup basketball games and intense workouts. I was meeting new people and starting my rigorous coursework as a nutrition science major. Once I got settled in, it was the same routine as it had been back in high school. I was waking up as early as the gym opened, after hearing my motivational song coming through my alarm. That meant it was time to get out there and put that work in, starting with my 6:30 am basketball workouts and afternoon weightlifting sessions. As soon as the alarm went off I was on the move, trying to make the most of every minute of my life. One big-time goal I had coming in was to walk on to the Cornell basketball team. I knew this would be a challenge, but I never accepted limits and always believed anything is possible and would do whatever it took. My high school AAU coach put in a good word to the Cornell coach, and I was going to work my butt off to be as ready as ever for a tryout. He suggested that I first try out for the club team as a way for me to inform the Cornell coach how I matched up against other top players at the school. Now, keep in mind that at a D1 school, there are a lot of great athletes who don't play for the varsity teams. So, the tryout consisted of many D3 and maybe even some D2 level players. When tryouts started, it felt as if everything was in slow motion and all was moving in my favor…I didn't miss a shot the entire tryout. I made 11/11 three pointers, and every time I shot the ball the other players would yell out "cash" or "money," and then splash, nothing but net. I called my parents that night to let them know about how incredible the tryout went.

9

This was all happening 3 weeks into my first ever college semester. It seemed that all of my years of dedication and long hours of hard work in everything I set out to do was going to produce the results I wanted. At the time, I held the belief that sleep was time wasted, so I had to constantly be working. Then BOOM! It hit me like a freight train. Next thing I know I'm in a coma, intubated and on a ventilator with a feeding tube, unable to move and unable to speak at all...fighting for my life.

You're probably wondering how I got here.

REWIND BACK TO EARLY CHILDHOOD
Chapter 2

Born in Long Island, New York, August 17th, 1996 to my two wonderful parents Ellen and Philip Weiss. Also there to welcome me was my older brother. We lived in Plainview up until I was 2, when we moved to Jericho.

Like most kids, I loved playing with Power Rangers, Pokémon, and Yu-gi-oh too. I discovered early on that I had an obsession with sports, and whether it was a bouncy ball, a basketball, baseball, soccer ball, or a football, I needed to be holding a ball at all times. There's a great video of me from when I was around 3. I'm in the basement and there's a Fisher Price hoop nearby. I have a tiny basketball in my hands and am wearing a Chicago Bulls Jersey to represent my favorite player at the time, Michael Jordan. My mom, who's videotaping, says to me, "What do you want to do now?" And my immediate response was, "Play basketball!" as I proceed to dunk the ball on the mini hoop. Thus started my love for sports. Having my dad as a coach in every sport and my parents showing

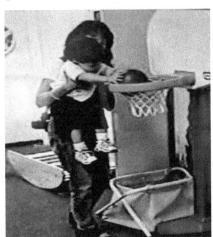 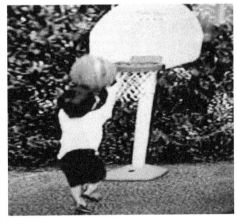

up to every single one of my games became a theme. I was always small in size, but I wouldn't let that stop me. I played basketball, baseball, soccer, and flag football. I was always super active. I have the most loving and caring parents in the world, and even though at times they can be strict and overprotective, they were always there for me and are my base and foundation. And I really can't complain because they shaped me into the amazing individual I am. This incredibly strong family connection will continue to be established throughout the book.

I went to nursery school and camp early on and loved it, as I was often having fun in the treehouse, and painting and playing with my friends. My best memory from camp was doing a dance to the Rolling Stones song "Satisfaction." Everyone in the group had to paint a letter on their chest and we all took our shirts off to show it off.

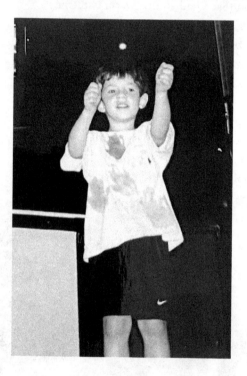
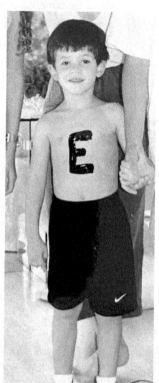

Camp consisted of swimming, karate, as well as a bunch of sports and crafts. All summer long, I anticipated the fun of Color War where groups would compete in games and sports.

When I turned 5, I attended elementary school. On the first day I recall being super nervous because I didn't know any kids. We all had name tags in the shape of apples, which quickly led to my meeting of two friends with whom I remained close throughout elementary school. While in kindergarten we had a new addition to my family as my little brother Brandon was born, which created huge excitement in our house. Our family had always been incredibly close, but Brandon really was the glue that we needed to solidify the family. My brothers were my best friends, and our family was extremely close. You'll understand later on why I like to say that when your family are your best friends and your best friends are your family, you know you have something special.

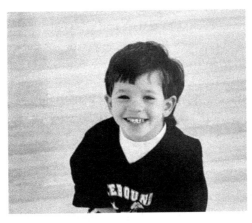

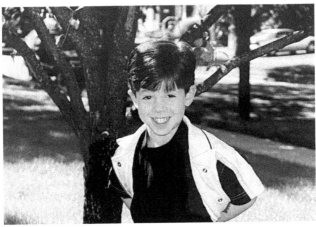

FAMILY

Chapter 3

My family is the most amazing base of support there could possibly be. Throughout the book, you'll hear me talk about how important my inner circle is to me, and that starts with my family.

Mom and Dad: My parents are the two most loving parents one could ever ask for. I know that no matter what they do, it's out of love. My dad has been my coach from day 1 no matter the sport. He has shown up to every game and every event I ever had, and worked with me at whatever it was I wanted to get better at, as well as taught me the value of consistent practice. Most importantly, he instilled in me that with hard work, anything is possible. And my mom has always been the kindest most loving mother ever, and there is nothing that she wouldn't do for her kids. She has always been my biggest supporter as well, encouraging me, as well as being the shoulder to cry on when I needed it most. I know that I can trust her with anything.

If I had to choose certain traits from my parents and tried to find where my personality came from (although there are many other events and life experiences that helped shape it outside of my parents as well), I would say my super competitiveness was instilled in me by my dad, as well as my striving to rise above the people who put me down. My love for doing things my way and my routine and insane work ethic probably comes more from my dad too. The part of me that tries to be the nicest person and never wants to hurt anyone, as well as my sensitivity, comes from my mom. In addition, being a perfectionist and also someone who takes things literally probably comes from my mom as well. Both parents taught me to always strive for greatness in everything that I do and taught me that no matter how small I am to always dream big because I can make an impact in the world.

My Brothers: They were the first best friends I was given. My older brother is 2 years older than I, and he has always defended me when I needed it and has been there to support me through it all. Of course just like any brother we have fought a lot over the years, but we would always fight for each other when it came down to it. Brandon is almost 6 years younger than I, and we are super close. We cheer each other on and cheer each other up and are the best teammates whenever we're together. I know whenever I need a fun time and something to take my mind off of the difficult times, he has always been there whether it be playing showdown cards, video games, basketball, low rim dunk contests, nok hockey, ping pong etc. And I can always count on him to be the first person to like my social media posts as he is my most loyal fan. Even on the occasional post where I would get only 1 or 2 likes, I know he'll be the one, which is one big factor that encouraged me to keep posting! We have spent years talking about serious and not so serious things. My brothers and I are all each other's biggest fans.

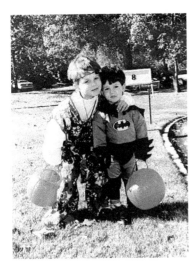
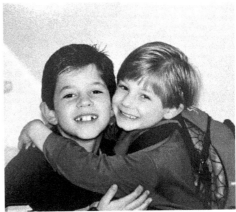

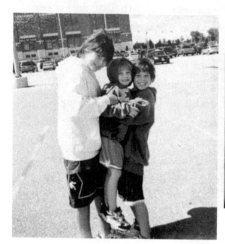
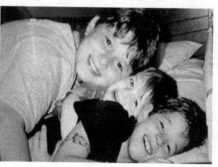
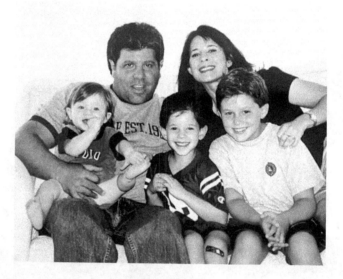

Jared Weiss

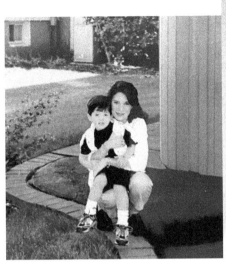

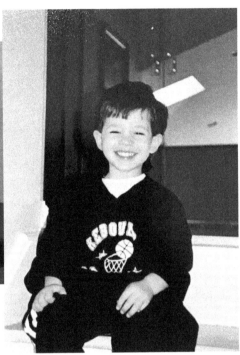

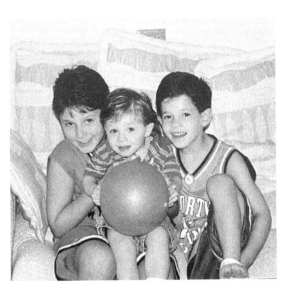

ANXIETY
Chapter 4

The first manifestations of separation anxiety were starting up early on in elementary school. My mom would come in to help with a class project or read to the class, and as soon as she left I would begin sobbing incessantly. Some mornings I wouldn't even get on the school bus. My dad would drive me to school and talk to me outside the classrooms until I was finally ready to go in. Up until middle school, there would be times where if I even thought about my family not being with me, I would get horrible anxiety and start crying. This also translated to playdates and practices. It was becoming a bit of an issue. I would get extremely upset and nervous when either I was at a friend's house, or when there were a bunch of kids at my friend's house on a playdate. A lot of people gathered together made me nervous. Oddly enough to this day, I still don't really like hanging out in big groups of people. I was always extremely sensitive, which at that time in my life I had seen as a weakness. Yet, being so sensitive and having this anxiety at a young age helped me learn a lot about understanding others and empathizing with them. Kids can be ruthless. Thankfully they weren't making fun of me for the crying, but rather they were always calling me names and commenting on how short I was, and really at times making me feel worthless. At the time I guess it was tough to see, but when others make fun of you it usually has nothing to do with you and means they are insecure. My parents constantly preached this.

My separation anxiety also carried over to other areas of my life. For instance at soccer tryouts when I was in 4th grade, if I didn't see one of my parents there at all times I would break out crying. Every time I lost sight of them I became extremely anxious. One time during the last tryout, when I was trying out for goalie, I ran off before it was over because I couldn't find my parents and had a little panic attack. My close friend's dad was right there with a water bottle, as he thought I was dehydrated and called my parents to come right away. The same occurred for everything; anytime I was out waiting for my parents to pick me up, they HAD to be exactly on time or else I would flip out and start hysterically crying. This lasted for a while. I have always had a strong attachment to the loved ones in my life.

SPORTS AS A METAPHOR FOR LIFE...
Chapter 5

You are going to hear me talk about sports a lot throughout the book, and even if you aren't super into sports or never played them, I feel that you can still find value in these chapters and let me explain why. So, first off sports have played a huge role in my life, but for me it wasn't always about the sports themselves, it was the lessons I learned from them. At times, I would get too caught up in tying my identity into how good I was or how good others thought I was, but now I see that tying your identity into how good of an athlete you are is dangerous because you can't directly control it and you can't control how others view you. Sports aren't everything. But they can be a really great metaphor for living life and this is why I fell in love with them at such a young age. These lessons I have learned set the stage for being able to conquer battles I would go onto face in my life later on. As with anything, to be your best, you have to work hard and work smart. There will be tons of failures and difficult losses that you will have to go through as well as the highs that come when you can put it all together and win. It takes a lot of researching and experimenting with various training methods, going through a lot of ups and downs, but staying with it will bring you farther than if you were to quit. Striving to be the best will take all you've got, yet still nothing is guaranteed. Just as with anything else in life, it's not always "fair" and sometimes you don't get the opportunities you deserve. Not every coach or teammate has your best interests at hand, so sometimes you may have to switch things up and go a different direction. You might get knocked down so hard that it feels you can't get up. But every time you do, you are proving to yourself what you are truly capable of. It's through these sports, as one of many avenues, that I like to show myself and others that anything is possible. Hopefully, these metaphors can be related to whatever it is that you are doing, so keep this in mind as you read on.

Note to the reader: The first few chapters in the book, you will notice how I make a number of references to details from my games when I talk about different scenarios and shots I took and scores of games. You may not be that interested in every minor detail, but just know that I am planting a foundation for you to understand my personality. This is to set the stage for how sports made me feel during those years as they played a huge role in my development. Learning about the intricacies of those games will provide you with a complete picture of how I internalized so much and how it all played out into making me who I am today.

Sports Early On

My dad always coached me and he coached me hard. Even when my dad wasn't "the coach" he's always been "my coach." He would often raise his voice as he was passionate and wanted me to be the best player, just as I wanted to be the best player. I may not have completely understood the spirit and affection behind it at the time, but the one thing I did always know was that he believed in me. Although this caused me a lot of internal anxiety to please him, it also motivated me and made me want to strive for more. More than anything, he wanted me to succeed and wanted me to prove to myself how good I was capable of becoming. He was (and still is) always working with me no matter the time of day. As I already mentioned, I played basketball, baseball, soccer, and flag football. In travel sports I started off making the B team in basketball, soccer, and baseball. I felt like I was an A team player, but wasn't good at asserting myself or taking charge, and to add to that I was always the shortest kid on the team. This required me to practice double time and really hone in all my skills.

Basketball Early Years

During those early years, I often lacked confidence in large part due to my being undersized. So, when coaches would see some of the bigger kids and say how great they were, that put a dent in how good I thought I could be. Also, I would get extremely nervous and had intense anxiety whenever games would come, and having to interact with kids I didn't know well made me uncomfortable. I would play really well when my dad was coaching me, and I definitely held my own during those years due to my dad's training and coaching me to ensure that I took my shots. I needed a coach and teammates who believed in me, but early on unfortunately I didn't have that outside of my dad. When the first travel team tryouts came along, I knew that my skills were A-team worthy, but being shy and nervous hurt me as I played a bit passively. I was way too unselfish and didn't realize that I wasn't going to be passed the ball unless I demanded it. I was never the type of kid who was loud enough to demand anything and felt bad about being selfish. Kids who I knew I was better than made the A team over me, and I made the B team. This hurt but also sparked a fire in me that would burn for years later anytime anyone doubted how good I could become at anything. All that work would eventually pay off, but the fire doesn't get lit without having our fair share of doubters, getting cut from teams, or being told we're not worthy of doing something enough times.

Soccer Early Years

Whereas basketball has always been my first love, soccer has been a close second. Early on, my dad used to enter a team into numerous indoor tournaments with me and my friends at the time. We had an awesome routine: wake up really early, sometimes go to New Jersey or to a bunch of local places, pick up my friend and his dad, as well as one or two other kids occasionally, then head to the indoor gym for a full day of soccer. I was the goalie. We won just about every tournament that we

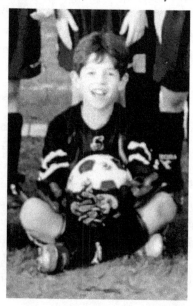

were in. However, in 4th grade I tried out for the travel team and made the B team as a field player. That first year, however, having some separation anxiety prompted me to transfer to the C team because this was the only way that my dad could coach me. At the time I was really fast and pretty good at ball handling. I started to develop a special toughness, which later on made me a perfect candidate to play goalie once again.

Soccer-5th grade

I moved up to the B team the following year for travel soccer. Then one day during halftime our goalie decided that he didn't want to play goalie anymore. The coach asked who wanted the position. My dad convinced me to volunteer. This was the start of an awesome revamped goalie career. For the next few years I manned the net. I felt like I controlled the game and the best thing was I wasn't going to be taken out by the coach. Strangely enough, as anxious a person as I was, I always enjoyed high pressure situations and positions in sports. Can't say I didn't get nervous leading up to these games, but as soon as it's a do or die situation, you could trust me to bring out my best. My dad would always be there standing on the sideline, talking to me during the game and coaching me, hard as always, but also cheering on every save I made. During one of these games, the ball was bouncing my way. My dad and teammates were frequently telling me to be more aggressive and come out of goal more often. If there was one flaw I had as a goalie early on, it was my fear of coming out and getting kicked, and boy did I ever. So the ball is bouncing my way and I run towards it, and as soon as I touch the ball, the kid running full speed kicks me in my mouth. To this day I have no idea how the ref didn't call a foul since I had the ball in my hands and the kid scored, and I'm on the ground in extreme pain. Somehow my dad drove me to go (you know how dads are) back into the game, and I later found that a piece of my tooth had come out of my mouth and onto my goalie gloves. That tooth is still slightly chipped to this day.

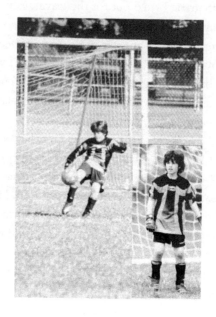

Baseball

Growing up I also loved playing baseball. Once again, my dad coached me. And I would go on to play travel baseball later on. I tried just about every position but mainly settled on 2nd base and outfield. I made the B team in travel baseball just as I had with the other sports, before working my way up to the A team. I also played summer ball, where we traveled to

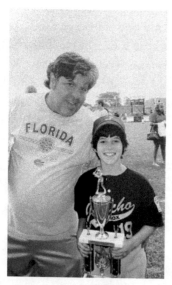

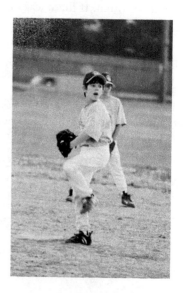

Massachusetts and competed in local tournaments and almost qualified for the Little League World Series. In middle school I finally started to hit my stride after years of training. Just 1 year removed from a summer where I had maybe 1 hit total, I had my best season in 7th grade where my friend and I had a competition to see who would win the team batting title…we each hit over .700 that year! That's the thing though, you never know when your breakthrough is coming, but that's why you can't quit on yourself. However, after my 8th grade year, it became completely unworkable to be present at every game and every practice I had. It was hard enough playing 3 different sports in a day at times and changing in the car and going from game to game. As much as I loved playing baseball, I wasn't as passionate as I was about my other sports. All of the sports began to conflict and it came down to the time when I had to choose. I didn't want to give up any of them, but I also couldn't keep missing games and practices, so by freshman year I had to give up baseball. I still ended up with 3 other sports which wasn't typical, but I couldn't stop!

Flag Football

The one other sport I played that I have yet to mention was flag football. This was super fun and very low stress, even though my dad, as always, loved to yell and coach us hard. My team won two Super Bowls in all of the years playing and we enjoyed those games tremendously. Especially the one that we played in 10 degree weather where our quarterback was still throwing bombs to me and two of my teammates. At halftime my friend and I had to sit in his dad's car just to warm up. *Me being the crazy kid I am, I wore shorts to that game!* My whole family came to the game as per usual, all bundled up and cheering me on.

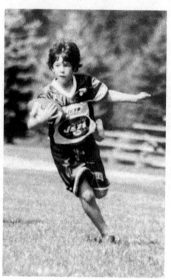

(This is from one of my early years playing flag football)

CHILDHOOD AWAKENING...NOT EVERYONE IS AS NICE AS YOU

Chapter 6

Growing up I had my fair share of bullies. I think most people deal with them at one point or another so I'm not gonna say my experience was totally unique, but it definitely contributes to shaping who you are. Like I said I was always a super nice kid, very sensitive, was short, and most likely not gonna fight back. Kids saw me as someone who they could easily pick on. It's weird how that works. They knew I would never do anything to hurt any of their feelings, so why would they do this to me? This was an early but powerful life lesson about people. This brings me to another story...Around 90% of the kids who my dad had coached absolutely loved him. He brings more intensity and passion than anyone. He is more vocal than anyone when you do something wrong, but will also cheer the loudest when you do something right and make you feel on top of the world. Some kids just couldn't handle this intensity, and at times I have felt the same way. But, I never thought anyone would talk bad about my dad behind my back because I would never have done that to anyone else. One day, when I was in 6th grade sitting at the lunch table, I overhear kids badmouthing my dad and saying how he takes coaching too seriously and how they don't like playing for him. And the one leading the talks was supposed to be my best friend. I didn't even know what to say. I came home crying to my mom that day. I felt betrayed, and as I discovered this wouldn't be the first time either.

In my family we don't let others get bullied without us having a say in it. Around the same time, I was dealing with one bully in particular who just wouldn't leave me alone and I needed some help. I saw the kid in school and sports practices and games and he just continued making fun of me. Then, we were at the same event, and he started up with me again. That night must've been the scariest night of his life. First, my older brother and his friends called him out and started roughing him around. Then, later on my mom found him and laid into him like you wouldn't believe, especially since my mom is the sweetest person in the world. But if you mess with her kids, you're gonna hear from her. That kid never spoke to me again after that night. That's what it means to be part of a family though, knowing they have your back and you have theirs. Whenever any of my friends early on in my life would get made fun of, I always stepped in and would stick up for them as best I could. Like the time when I pushed a kid down at camp because he kept pushing my friend. Or the time in 5th grade when two of my friends were arguing and one insulted the other's dad whom I loved, and I let him know that he crossed the line. My parents always taught me that you have to stick up for yourself because if not, you're just gonna keep getting pushed around. As the years went on I got better at speaking up for and defending myself as uncomfortable as it is, but sometimes it's necessary. And same goes for my friends today-if you mess with them, you gotta deal with me (although of course it's best to first try to deescalate every situation if possible). I will always have their backs and when they're hurting that affects me deeply. And thankfully I have a team of family and friends behind me that I know I can trust to do the same for me, as they always have.

I now realize that it is actually you who gives these bullies power, because when you show that you don't care what they are doing and you are not going to change your behaviors, then you take back control. And moreover, whenever possible just get these people out of your life because they're only gonna be draining your energy. Today, I have real friends and family and we have each others' backs. It wasn't always like that and it takes constantly reforming and reshaping your circle to get it right. People sometimes make fun of you and try to lower you because they know they can, and they feel that it raises them. Make sure that your circle is full of people who want the best for you and want to see you win!

Jared Weiss

CAMP...MY HAPPY PLACE
Chapter 7

The summers would soon become my favorite time of the year, as day camp was my favorite place on Earth. This was my happy place. There were so many incredible counselors and super fun activities at this wonderful camp. It was full of sports and swimming and friends and people who were encouraging me to just be myself and have fun. Time was occupied every second of the day. Plus there were so many awesome competitions which fed right into my competitive nature, such as Olympics and Color War. We had a blast. This was where I first learned that it's not about what you're doing but who you're doing it with that can turn an ordinary experience into a valuable memory. When I first started, the camp wasn't in the best condition, but it never mattered to me. As I got older I would have to convince my friends to keep coming back. They would complain that the camp was falling apart and that they would rather go to a nicer camp. But I would ask them, "Has the condition ever stopped us from having the best time?" It truly never even occurred to me that the camp wasn't being kept up, and I think this speaks to who I am today. I don't need a lot to be happy and have fun. I don't mind things that are simple. Oftentimes the simplest times are the best, and it's the people who you spend them with that matters. As I became a preteen and teen, I started the travel program, which was unnerving the first year since I didn't like to be away from my parents. One summer, I met with a psychologist to help me get over my fears. It was a slow process, but I persevered and went on the overnight trips and had a blast, in spite of the first few where I was extremely homesick. On one of the first overnight trips, suddenly I became overwhelmed with feelings of homesickness right after speaking to my parents. My friends who were in my hotel room decided to ask for their names and act like my family members. This gave me a good laugh and made me feel a bit more comfortable. I loved my counselors and developed special relationships with them, just as I would with my campers when I became a counselor years later. I always preferred the camp people to the school people because the camp itself fostered an environment where I could be my true self and come out of my shell. I had a lot more confidence and typically less anxiety when I was there. The people there got to know the real me and see me in my best light. In school I often felt constrained while being told to sit down and listen to what the teachers had to say. Also, school tends to lead to cliques being formed, and being forced to fit in and do the same thing as everyone else made me uncomfortable. Camp friendships always seemed to come easier and be more meaningful. Little did I know how much this place would eventually mean to me as an oasis for my emotional health, and little did I know that my future best friends would come from this place.

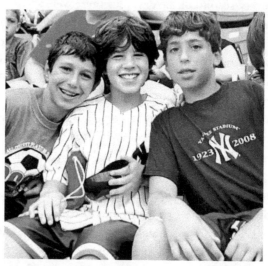

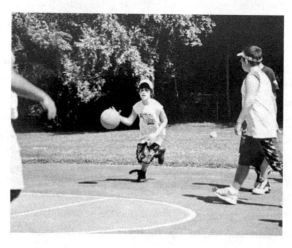

THE MIDDLE SCHOOL YEARS-CREATING SOME DISTANCE

Chapter 8

Between the years of 6th through 8th grade I started off with what I thought was a good amount of friends. I was always very optimistic and figured these people were all my real friends; however, slowly something began to change. In middle school there was a very difficult change of pace. I was super nervous and recall crying on the first day, missing my family and not wanting to be in this new place. Soon after, I met some new kids from the other elementary schools and found my way. By 7th grade, school sports started and I was playing basketball, soccer, baseball, as well as flag football. I didn't have a ton of confidence around others though. I was often afraid that others didn't like me. I started to become a perfectionist and really worked hard to please my parents. I never wanted to disappoint them or mess up. The only real trouble I ever got into would be talking in class while the teacher was talking, or driving my brothers crazy by annoying them with singing, or trying to get their attention while we were supposed to be doing homework. I began to learn how I loved to work hard and loved that people thought I was smart. It's sort of like a positive feedback loop where the more your peers tell you that you're good at something, the harder you want to work to prove them right. This started to feed into my work ethic and competitive desire to set high goals.

Then came the bar and bat mitzvah years and this played a large role in social life at the time in my hometown. At many of these bar/bat mitzvah parties, I started to see a pattern. Even at that young age, most people were more concerned about being popular than they were being with a true friend. It was all about "who can I hang out with at this party to make me look more popular and cool?" I was invited to just about all of the parties, but the kids who I thought were my friends a lot of times left me by myself. And I never wanted to be a follower, so I learned early on that I would rather be by myself than with others who didn't want me around. Being shy and uncomfortable at parties in general didn't help my case, but I figured if you want to talk to and hang with me I'd be happy to, but I'm not gonna chase and follow you around to be your friend. My own bar mitzvah happened to be an incredible time and an awesome accomplishment. After all the practice everything went smoothly and the party was amazing. My dad knew a guy who worked with rappers and performers, so I was able to get a rapper named Ron Browz to come and perform a few songs. (His major hit song was "Pop Champagne" and he's also a big-time producer). It was nice to finally feel like I was the star of the show.

By the end of middle school, I was becoming more independent and just loved working out and playing my sports, always putting work into improving myself, whether it be in the gym or in my studies. I also absolutely loved reading tons of books and gaining new knowledge on a variety of topics that interested me. The kids around me were really changing and I didn't like who they were becoming, so I started to create distance between me and them.

Basketball-Middle School

In 6th grade, a blessing of a coach came my way. His name was Ritchie Gabriel. I was trying out for an AAU team at the time but the team folded and Ritchie decided to coach my travel team. My dad also hired him to train me. For the first time, I really felt like a coach believed in me, aside from my dad, and he wanted me to succeed more than anything else. He always told me to keep shooting the ball, stop being so unselfish and told me the team needed me to win. The start of that season was like the prior one. I knew what I could do, but was hesitant to put my skills to use and was plagued by anxiety. Then, in one game, our hardest of that season, versus a top team, everything just clicked in me. I took my first 3 pointer of the season, top of the key....*SWISH*. Five more threes like that and a team who should've beaten us by 30 only won by single digits. Ritchie was proud of me, my parents as always were proud of me, and for once I had a sliver of confidence myself. Once I showed myself what was possible, I realized how good I could be. The next game I had 17 points and made the game tying shot at the buzzer to go into overtime. I had 2 more game winners during that year as well. It was a turning point in my athletic

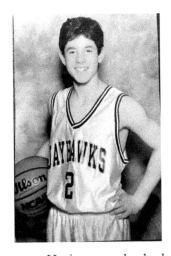 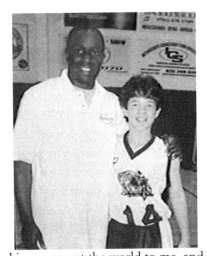

career. Having a coach who believed in me meant the world to me, and sometimes that's all it takes. A great coach, mentor, or role model in general can seriously change a kid's or anyone's life. The next year I was asked to play on the A team, but I chose to stick with my new favorite coach. We formed our own AAU team with some top notch players, and soon after I was being asked to play for other AAU teams. In 8th grade, I went on to play for the LI Kings coached by a new friend, Omar, along with his son Tyree who I met at Island Garden basketball camp. I also had a new favorite teammate in Elisha. He and I connected first on Ritchie's team and both of us went to this Kings team with Omar. Elisha was the slasher and dunker and high flyer, and I was the trusted outside shooter who he could always count on to nail a 3. I loved playing with Elisha because he gave me the confidence I needed from a teammate, as he always made it known that he was trusting me to knock down the shots and would tell me to keep my head up whenever I missed. Having teammates who maintain trust in you to take the next shot even when you're missing is invaluable and rare to find, and this goes for anything, not just sports. We played in places like Far Rockaway, the Bronx, New Jersey and all over the Northeast. Once we even had to go home before a game because a kid on the other team had been shot beforehand. This was a very unsettling and eye opening experience. It was hard for me to process. Occasionally we would stop at places like Burger King for lunch in the interest of time. Since I was the only one trying to eat healthy, I would order the grilled chicken, which drew many laughs from my coach and teammates.

Basketball-AAU-high school

After excelling in some tough tournaments, I was asked to play for the Unique All Stars coached by NBA player Tobias Harris's father Torrell Harris. This was the highest level of AAU ball there was. Let me start by saying that you don't know how tough a coach can be until you play for Torrell. He had a booming voice which reverberated throughout the empty gym where we practiced. Our one reprieve was every once in a blue moon, Torrell would teach us dance moves to practice our shiftiness on the court. But, truth be told, he was the hardest coach to play for in the world. Those practices were tougher than ever. Not gonna lie, he made my already bad anxiety even worse, and it skyrocketed. Whenever we had a practice my stomach would start to turnover a thousand times and my whole body would tense up. If the offensive player made a really nice move and scored, the defensive player would be told how bad he did even if the shot was heavily contested. We ran endless suicides every time our scrimmage team lost. Postgame conferences were not fun and sometimes we even got singled out in front of everyone. All of this disciplining for poor play also led to teammate fighting, which made me more upset than anyone. I'm not a confrontational person and I hate fighting with others. Me being someone who never likes to blame others, I would just take it and not give it. It was not all bad though. I remember my first game with this team was pretty awesome but it all happened in a blur. The first few practices had gone really well for me, and the players seemed to like my unselfishness and that I was a good shooter. So, we were down by a few points about midway through the first half when Coach puts me in after screaming at the kid who he took out. The first play, I hit a 3 (I still have no idea how that shot went in). I was so afraid of Torrell yelling at me, but I threw the ball up and somehow it swished. Then, next possession I shut down my guy on defense, got a steal and an assist and another assist the play after, giving us the lead and turning the momentum of the game over. My nickname became Nash. This was a great honor to me considering that my favorite pro player was Steve Nash. Since 2004-2005 when I was 8 years old I was so inspired by the point guard for the

Phoenix Suns (Steve Nash). He won 2 MVP awards, although if you saw him you wouldn't think he's a basketball player. He played without fear

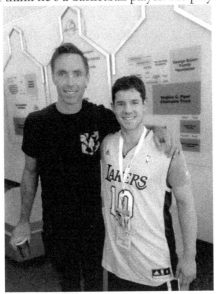

and his skill was unmatched. I bought some of his training DVDs. I wanted to know everything about him, and he was showing me that it's possible for someone like me to excel in basketball. I even had my hair like his for a while as well. And then in 2015, thanks to my family friends who knew a trainer that used to work with his former team, I was even lucky enough to meet him!

Torrell didn't compliment often, but when he did you felt on top of the world. Like at this tournament in Lefrak City when I had the game winning steal and assist, Torrell called my dad up afterward telling him that I was going to be just like Steve Nash and that I was gonna play college ball. Then, there was the time when he made me a starter after telling kids who were 2 years older than me that I was a much better player than they were. Or at our tournament at Elmcor in 10th grade when I was scoring really well and I was almost awarded MVP of the tournament. Also, when our team went to Boo Williams and then Florida, Torrell was so impressed with my defense as I shut down the best guards on a few different teams. Torrell commended my effort so passionately and told me that I was going to be able to play in the Ivy League. We traveled all around the country with this team. And he respected my hard work and effort. Moreover, at the end of my 2nd year with the team, we had an awards ceremony and there were a bunch of small trophies and only 3 big ones. Torrell goes through every player on the team and gets down to the 2nd to last award with just 2 huge trophies left and my name yet to be called. He announces this tremendous trophy, the "Most Courageous Player" award, and says Jared Weiss. There was a mix of good

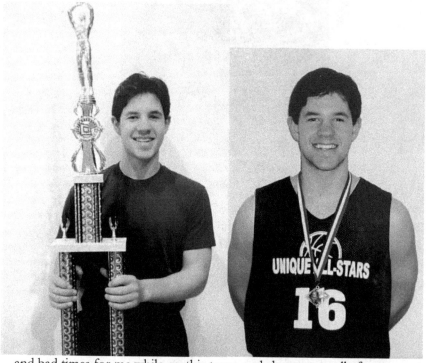

and bad times for me while on this team, and also some really funny times. One such time was when I had an outdoor tournament and I was starting off on the bench. Some guy walks by and starts shouting so everyone could hear, "Put the white boy in!"

There was also one game, probably one of the only games ever that neither of my parents was in attendance for. Torrell drove me. And midway through the game, I pump faked, drove the ball into the paint and ran into a 6'8 guy's shin or knee I believe and my eye was gushing blood. Omar and Elisha were in attendance for this game so they came to check on me as I went to the bathroom to try to put a towel on my eye. Then on the way home I start to get a headache. Torrell tried to call my parents to tell them what happened and they started freaking out. They had no clue what to expect and Torrell wasn't even sure of the severity of this yet. The headache worsened and my parents took me to the hospital and I found out I had a concussion. You can imagine how scared my mom was. After that, for the next few years my mom made me wear a mouthguard and a goalie helmet whenever I played goalie in soccer (the one Peter Czech used to wear). I don't think my parents missed another game since then lol.

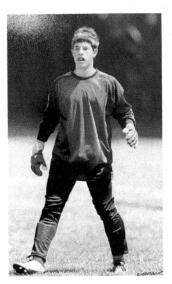

But this style of coaching was not helping my confidence much. It might have worked for others, but it wasn't working for me. The constant back and forth between scoldings and only seldom receiving compliments was not allowing my game to progress. My self-esteem was taking hits day by day, and I'm a player who works off of confidence. If I don't have that then I can't play up to my best. I'm already hard enough on myself and tend to overthink everything. I finally reached the point when I knew that it was time to get back to playing MY game. One of the hardest things as an athlete is playing for a coach who you're afraid is going to take you out after every little mistake. Unfortunately, I played for a lot of these coaches and in some ways that shaped my performance anxiety. I spoke with my dad and told him that I could be doing so much more as a player if only I

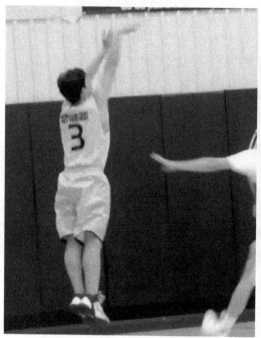
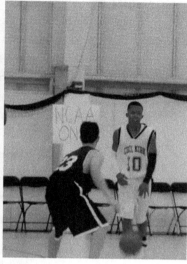

had the right system where I was being encouraged rather than broken down. Ironically, within weeks after leaving both AAU teams, the teams broke up, but I eventually reconnected and maintained good relationships with those coaches because I was able to take what I learned from these experiences and use them constructively to grow as a player. Torrell is one of my dad's best friends. My dad works with him as well, and these days when I see him he is so kind and encouraging towards me. And Omar would go on to train me throughout high school, while Tyree and Elisha would play on several of my new teams. As you'll see later on Omar also played a monumental role in my initial recovery process. We decided it was time for me to reunite with my favorite coach, the one who helped me fall in love with the game and believed in my potential. Ritchie, along with my dad, would coach me in tournaments until the end of high school, and my scoring as well as my overall performance was able to flourish again. I wasn't afraid to shoot or to mess up, and I was able to add that to my intense full court defense attack instilled in me by my prior coaches. I also played for some other high-quality teams such as with Coach Warren and Coach Barry, as well as lower pressure CYO and PAL teams during this time too with Coach Dan; it was a good fit between those coaches and me. I think sometimes we forget why we play these games when we take them so seriously. We need to remind ourselves how sports are supposed to be fun, and that's what teams like those did for me as these were some of my favorite times playing basketball. School basketball is a whole other story which I will get into later…

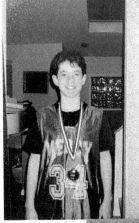

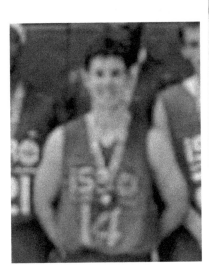
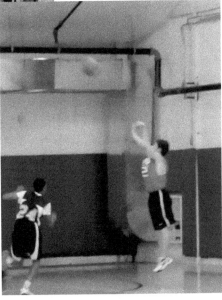

Nutrition Interest-Middle School

When I was in 6th grade, my friend's cousin was in from Florida and we went to a diner after a travel basketball game. I always had so much respect and admiration for those who have a lot of knowledge to offer. So when he started talking about the importance of nutrition for athletic performance, I was all ears. Now keep in mind he was not saying that you couldn't eat junk food for the rest of your life or that you had to always eat healthy…or else, but me being the literal person I am took it 100% literally. Some may argue that I took it too far, but shortly after this time was when I began searching for every competitive advantage I could get, so upgrading my diet made sense. These major dietary changes wouldn't happen for a few years though. Anyways the conversation was very interesting as he proceeded to tell me how eating healthy makes you a better athlete and helps people function more efficiently. When the bar/bat mitzvahs started up in 7th grade I ate so much candy (I know…hard to believe for all of you who know me now lol). After I ate the candy I would estimate how many calories I had eaten, come home and go in my bathroom do 10 sit-ups and 10 pushups for every 100 calories of junk food I thought I ate. Maybe it was a borderline eating disorder but I didn't know any better. To make matters a bit worse, one day at the lunch table one of my friends was showing everyone how skinny he was. He had always been that way as that was his body type, really thin and had small bones, but this made me think that I had some weight to lose even though I had always been in good shape, and if anything I was on the skinny side. I thought this was a good time to apply the knowledge that I had learned from my friend's cousin.

Unfortunately I didn't have guidance on how to go about it at first, so this led to some pretty uneducated and dangerous habits. I was exercising for hours a day trying to burn as much body fat as possible. I was drinking tons and tons of water and looking at how many calories were in every food I ate. When I wasn't doing calisthenics or weight training I would use the treadmill because that told me how many calories I had burned. I had good intentions of trying to be healthy, but I just had no clue how to do it safely. I did tons of nutrition research and took every statement to the max. When I would read about vitamins being good for you I would try to get as many as possible. For instance, I would have a bowl of cereal, usually *Total*, thinking that was great for me because they advertised how many vitamins were in there (I didn't understand the difference between fortified vs vitamins from foods). Another favorite of mine was *Special K* since the commercials spoke about weight loss (even though I didn't have any weight to lose). I wouldn't even have a full steak because I was afraid of gaining weight, so I would only have a few bites. In my mind, I thought calories were bad and would make me fat. But, meanwhile I was an athlete and training hard. So, these were not healthy behaviors. Also, one of my friends at the time was trying to lose weight to get himself healthy, so I would listen to him and that made me want to do what he was doing. I wouldn't even eat a full fruit cup for fear of eating too much sugar. My energy wasn't good and I was losing weight that I didn't have to lose. I would go to sleep hungry and tell my parents that I wouldn't eat more until I got a trainer.

Thankfully this only lasted for a short time and thank goodness for Michael Phelps. Yes, you read that right. The Olympic gold medal swimmer was getting really popular around this time, and I read an article about how he ate 10,000 calories a day to fuel his activities, but somehow he was really muscular. He mentioned how important it is for athletes to eat enough to fuel rigorous training. Then I thought to myself, why do I want to lose weight (including muscle) if all the best athletes are jacked? I would much rather get muscular to help my game. I started eating a lot more, still focusing on healthy food and working out a lot, but now I wasn't counting calories. I was trying to put on pounds of muscle to make others notice. And they did. Within a few months I had a solid 6 pack of abs and toned arms. I still had my big yet muscular legs, and I was at a healthy weight. My peers started to become impressed. They were saying how jacked I was and telling their friends to check out my abs and asking me to pop my pecs like Dwyane the Rock Johnson. They were asking what I was doing for my routine. My first true experience with lifting weights was when I joined my friend in the Strength and Conditioning after-school program at my school in 8th grade. I immediately fell in love. I felt like this was a place where I belonged.

Working out became my new hangout:

One reason why I loved going to the gym and continuing with basketball, soccer, and track is that I could work on improving my skills by myself. I am able to retreat into my own world. As I approached the end of middle school and beginning of high school I realized that I was often ending up alone. I was being left out by the kids that I was once comfortable with, and quite frankly I didn't want to participate in a lot of what they were doing. I told myself that I was too busy working towards my goals, and I didn't have time. I was definitely super busy all the time and I did enjoy my independence. And I think being comfortable and able to create happiness while alone is a very valuable skill to have, especially when that is the best option. Because when you are able to be happy while alone, you won't ever have to settle for others who aren't right for you. But having said that, truthfully, I really just didn't feel comfortable being myself around many of the other kids. As much as I enjoyed my own company and loved being with my family, I could've used some real friends at the time too, even though I told myself I didn't need anyone. So, I became obsessed.

You don't need an invitation to grind or work on yourself. Therefore, whenever I became sad or depressed or angry, I knew and still know today I could always count on the gym, because like I said all I needed was me, myself, and I. I find solace in the gym. You might be wondering how could I feel lonely when I was playing on all these sports teams and involved with all these other activities? Yes, I was interacting with others during the games, but I wasn't connecting with these kids outside of the games and practices. I always had my family to count on, but outside of that, the weights, the basketball, and the books were my best friends until I found the right people later on.

Everyone in the weight room was trying to get bigger, stronger, and faster just like me. I had lifted a couple of weights in my house in the past with my dad and brother, but I was mostly doing bodyweight training consisting of jump rope, sit-ups, pushups, and I was crafting my own routines. Some days I would go to the school weight room, and on others

42

I would do my own thing. Soon enough, I started combining the two… in addition to my sports training.

I wanted to get every workout program and piece of equipment known to man, starting with Perfect Pushup and Perfect Sit-up, yoga, stretching and athletic programs-Insanity and Insanity the Asylum and P90X. And my family's personal favorite (which they will never let me live down), the shake weight. This is what I would spend my birthday money on and what I would tell my friends and family whenever they asked what I wanted for my birthday. Then came the vertical jump programs, and I bought a lot of them, everything from the platform shoes to every program that promised to add 10 inches to my vertical jump and 20 pounds of muscle and whatever else they promised in a 1 month time period… The truth is they weren't all 'bad,' but I was so determined to better myself in any way possible that I was also naive enough to believe all of the exaggerated marketing claims. And I didn't have the knowledge and research to see that a lot of the programs were gimmicks not backed by any real results. Furthermore, I bought every basketball training program that promised to add 20 points to my scoring average and give me the best skills ever. My desire for self-improvement pushed me to look for tools to get better in every area of my life. Also, keep in mind that I was overworking my body to the max, as I didn't know enough about Central Nervous System (CNS) fatigue among many other aspects of overall health. I thought that more was always better. Unfortunately, it takes some trial by fire for people like me. It's a miracle that my body didn't actually fall apart. I really was trying to be the best…in everything. This is where addiction to improvement and success is a gift and a curse. Trying to become the best at everything takes a toll on your body and your mind. You get anxious and overthink things and make too much of what others are gonna think of you, and you start overworking and it can make you crazy. So, yes maybe I was a little crazy, but that's what fueled my drive.

Achieving this positive recognition for the work I was putting in made me happy. Yet there were other kids who called me crazy. They would say how hard of a worker I was and call me a "try hard." I took this as a compliment, and this made me want to reach as high as I could with everything I did. The harder I worked, the more it made me want to keep working hard. I became addicted to the grind. I loved chasing after my dreams.

Jared Weiss

HIGH SCHOOL-TAKING MY WORK ETHIC TO AN INHUMANE LEVEL

Chapter 9

As someone who tends to take everything literally, this made me a bit of a "crazy" person in high school. I started watching tons of motivational videos: Eric Thomas, Tony Robbins, Kobe Bryant, Les Brown. These people started to shape my thought patterns. I soon became a hyper motivated machine. I began playing for a wide variety of basketball teams outside of school, taking the hardest AP classes, and putting in more work and effort into everything I did. "The way you do anything is the way you do everything" is a quote that I still stand by to this day, so I'm not gonna say that going 1000% full force into everything was completely a bad thing. It definitely helped accomplish many goals, gave me a never back down and never give up mindset, and made me a relentless worker. But the one thing I didn't understand was the importance of rest and balance, and I think I could've accomplished just as much and probably more, in a healthier way had I understood this. I have no regrets because I learned through experience, although since hindsight is always 20-20, I would tell my past self that being a smart worker is more important than just being the hardest worker. However, that's why it's so important to continuously learn as you embark on this journey of life. Everyone's "balance" is different. **So what might be seen as doing too much for some people might be just right for you and vice versa, but it's up to you to always be in tune with your body and understand what your capacity for every endeavor is.** And if you are always ignoring what your body is telling you, this will get you into trouble. Although I didn't know at the time that what I was doing was not the best way, this was the only way I knew. **Also, I would later come to realize that the happier you are and the more fun you are having, the better you play and better you perform.** Sleep is so much more important than I was treating it. I thought that I was being the healthiest person because of my diet and workouts, however, sleep is instrumental to making your body work. Health is all about balancing mind, body, and spirit which includes having great friendships and developing these, and giving your body down time

45

which is imperative for overall success. Moreover, early on I didn't really understand the concept of diminishing returns. If I could get the same grade studying for 2 hours as I could for 6 hours, then those additional 4 hours can actually hurt me by essentially frying my brain, and same goes for my workouts.

There was always a chip on my shoulder to prove doubters wrong, so this lent itself to working inhumane amounts to do everything possible. I let my ego get the best of me sometimes and would push beyond what I was physically capable of at that moment. "No days off" for me literally meant no days off, no hours off, no time to relax-which I know now is 100% necessary for kids and anyone working towards their goals. I had to do everything my way and if I crashed, I would have to figure out the consequences on my own because I've never liked being told what to do. I figured that if I worked as hard as possible at everything then nobody could ever say I didn't do my best, even if I failed at what I was attempting. I thought this was what I HAD to do in order to achieve my goals of being the best athlete and student and hardest worker ever. I considered downtime to be laziness, so I thought occupying every waking minute would make me the best. My typical daily schedule by junior year had become wake up at 6 am to workout with my trainer, go to school from 8 am (usually club meetings or extra help before class) till 3:30 pm, then play whatever school sport was that season. I was on 3 varsity sports teams, one for every season from 4:15 until 6:15. Many nights my dad would come with me to put up extra shots or do extra reps of my sport. Most seasons I would also go to another practice for a team outside of school, then come home to study and do homework and sometimes have a tutor come, and finish with everything at about 2 to 3 in the morning on average. If I didn't understand every last detail or memorize every page in the textbook, my work was not complete. Keep in mind that I had numerous goals in all of the sports I played, but I didn't realize that proper rest would make me a better athlete. I would walk around school like a zombie. My body was shot. A few times per year I would get severe migraines as well as severe eye strain. It's a mystery that I was even able to perform the way I was considering the stress I would put my body through. The desire for greatness will push you to do some crazy things. I will reiterate here: my intentions were amazing and pushing your limits and working hard is necessary in order to be your best self, however this was taking things too far and was not healthy!

As I mentioned, I am a perfectionist and am thorough to a fault; I won't stop anything until I'm confident that I understand it completely. I've always been an extremely literal person; for instance if you tell me that fiber is good for you, I'll have 100 grams of it per day, or if you tell me that running is good I'll run as much as possible until I pass out. I guess most people understand not to take everything to the nth degree, but then again I'm not most people. There is a lot of false information out there that makes it hard for a kid to understand, especially one who takes everything so literally. (This is why I'm not good at understanding sarcasm and I'm typically the last one to get a joke).

Sacrifices are necessary to be the best version of yourself, but make sure you're sacrificing the right things. Although I unwisely sacrificed my sleep, I did achieve a ton of success by working as hard as I did. Heck, by the end of high school I was given the award of scholar athlete by having my high GPA to go along with three varsity sports letters. I got into an Ivy League school and was offered to play college basketball at a few D3 schools, one college track offer and a college soccer look. So while I did achieve many goals, my body certainly paid the price. There was not enough rest and downtime and I was not looking at my health from a holistic standpoint. Ironically, maybe this strong mindset was what got me through my tremendous health struggles later on. I wasn't out partying and never drank or smoked, never gave into peer pressure, and wasn't wasting time with people who I didn't like and those who weren't real friends. Yes, I should've been better at balancing and resting and understanding all the improvements I would ultimately make, but the only way to learn is through experience. That's why I'm telling you this stuff now, so that you don't have to go through it and can make wiser decisions and can respect and enjoy the process of reaching your goals.

Even to this day I still have to get better at knowing when to reign in my crazy work ethic and knowing when to take a break, and this would become a huge factor in my healing process too. It's not easy for me. Because in my mind, I always want to give everything my absolute all.

To be clear, this message is for the people who you have to hold back. I think we should all work as hard as we can, but part of that is knowing how much rest we need and allowing your body the chance to recover and improve because that's when the most gains happen. I'm all about the grind and this is what I preach. But part of the grind is knowing when to be smart and hold back. There were some people who tried to hold me back in order to stop me from causing damage to myself (like my mom) versus those who were trying to hold me back so I wouldn't get ahead of them. This is another important distinction to make. Know who's looking out for your best interests!

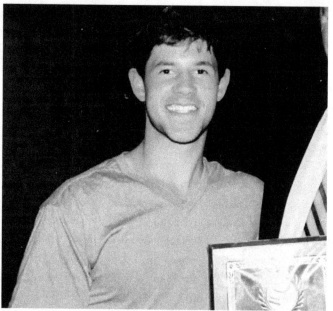

Accepting the scholar athlete award

ANYTHING IS POSSIBLE AND YOU COULDN'T CONVINCE ME OTHERWISE

Chapter 10

As a young kid I was always looking to try new things, constantly looking to experiment beyond what I had seen. When playing a sport it was trying out new moves or trying to jump as high as I could. I would often get laughed at whenever I would tell my friends that anything was possible. In spite of knowing what didn't seem possible, I had this unwavering belief in me that anything was possible and I would be able to reach anything I set my mind to. As cliché as this might sound, I still believe this to be true. The main reason we have doubt is because we allow ourselves to settle for mediocrity and close our minds off to the unseen. My parents would always tell me I was the best, yet I often felt I lacked confidence, especially in social situations. What I never lacked was a belief in my potential and what I was capable of doing and who I was capable of becoming. Part of confidence comes from how you think others view you and how you feel about yourself as a result, while self-belief is knowing what is possible. A high level of self-belief means knowing that you have unlimited potential. And when you realize how powerful we truly are as divine spiritual beings as I will get into later on, you will realize how we can manifest anything in our realities.

It takes a really long time and a lot of life experience to not care what others think about you. As much as we tell ourselves that we don't care, it is hard to fully believe it. Being told numerous times that you are too short and being called names starts to get to you after a while. Once I got to high school this served as my initial motivation to become everything they said I couldn't.

The doubters and the haters are sometimes what jumpstarts one's quest for prowess in any walk of life. Just look at Tom Brady, Michael Jordan, and Steve Jobs. If you listen to many of their interviews you begin to understand that their initial fuel and spark came from being told what they couldn't do, or a coach gave up on them, or a company went under.

So, after being cut from a few different teams, realizing how my height and my lack of "natural gifts" could be limiting factors, I continued my quest to become the best athlete possible and worked relentlessly towards this goal. Moreover, this would carry on into other aspects of my life such as academics. I wanted it all; I was driven to reach for the stars.

LIVING WITH NO LIMITS: TRYING TO ACHIEVE THE IMPOSSIBLE

Chapter 11

While striving to be the best student and the best athlete, people watching me in action often said to me that I must have really loved school. In reality that couldn't be farther from the truth. I've always been an optimistic and happy person, although it went against my grain to continually conform to the teachers' principles when I felt differently. It seemed like a waste of time to have to put in so many hours of studying material that I would never have to use again, only to vomit the information onto the test just to get a good grade. And then have to do it all over again. That system never felt right to me. But, I couldn't turn off the switch. That competitive nature, the drive, translates to everything I do. However, I was unable to have anticipated the hours upon hours this drive to achieve would take and all of the sacrifices in my life this would require. Yet I kept pushing and pushing and milking every last ounce of energy there was. I became used to feeling like my body was going to fall over at any point. There was just no off switch on me and you couldn't tell me otherwise. Once again, I accomplished a lot and am very proud of where my work ethic has led me. It's easy for me to see now that health isn't just eating healthy, not just working out all the time and having muscles, but it's also knowing when to give your body a REST. If you are anything like me and you have trouble stopping, know that you will pay for it one way or another.

Basketball-High School

In my mind you could be more talented than me, bigger and naturally more gifted, but you will not outwork me. As football player Ray Lewis once said, "Effort is between you and you." Nobody else can control your heart or determination but you. So, when high school sports started, it was the same thing. I would be sure to run harder, play harder defense, and do my best to always make the right play in all the sports I played. However, at this time, I had to choose certain sports teams based on when the games would not conflict. As I already mentioned, I still ended up with 3 sports throughout high school in addition to my outside of school teams (basketball, soccer and track), which is not typical, but I couldn't see myself parting with any of them. Oftentimes, I would have 3 sports on the same day and plenty of days were spent going from one sport or one team to the next, while changing and eating in the car, and finishing up the day late at night. I saw this as normal since I was so used to it over the years. But I didn't realize that putting all this pressure on myself to always perform at my best despite non-ideal conditions, and expecting an A in every class was a lot for a young kid to handle. Still, I never thought of this as impossible.

I tried out for the JV basketball team. I know that I was really small but that didn't matter because I believed my skills were worthy. In my opinion, coaches will often take someone who they see as having more potential due to natural gifts, such as being tall, instead of the kid who is going to outwork anyone. I was already playing on a top AAU team where the competition was super high level and intense. So at the JV tryouts, myself and 4 other 9th graders tried out. I really played well. I felt I was 100% worthy of a spot on the team. I won all the sprint drills, knocked down my outside shots, and played hard defense. The first cuts came by, I made it past them. Then on the last day I was sent back down to the 9th grade team. I heard later that the varsity coach's reasoning for my not making the JV team was, "If he was a good player, a college level player, I would've heard about him." This stoked a fire in me. Motivation. The grind was in full pursuit. I truly believe that each time I was told no, the fire in me grew bigger and I knew what I had to do.

The coach of the 9th grade team was actually the same one who cut me from the A team years ago. He had actually offered me a spot on the A team once my game had started blossoming in 6th grade, but I didn't take the spot because I was content being coached by Ritchie. He would also coach me in AAU a bit later on. Incidentally, by this point he had started coaching my brother Brandon and loved him as he was his star player. So anyway, the first day of practice comes and Coach Warren says to me, "I know how upset you are about not getting picked for the JV team. So prove to me that you deserved it. Make them regret that decision." I really appreciated that and felt like he understood me. I enjoyed playing for him and knew that he wanted the best for me. Occasionally I would get pulled for missing a shot and he was tough, but for the most part he let me play my game and believed in me. I worked my butt off and was a top player and top scorer on the team. Then, 10th grade rolls around and I make the JV team. Still small, but ferocious. When people or players told me I can't, I would say, "Watch me" and get to work. That year was definitely a great learning experience. In spite of being a top scorer on my team the year prior, the JV coach thrust me into a new role. First game of the season and I was coming off the bench as a 6th man. I came in and made all the right decisions as point guard, as well as played the best defense of my life and guarded pretty much every area of our matchup zone. After the game, the coach announced to the whole team that I was the reason why we won and he said that was exactly why I was coming off the bench, to provide a spark. I was upset about not starting but I embraced my role as a workhorse and an unselfish player.

Funny story…one practice I went for someone's pump fake and fouled them on the way down. Coach screams at me, "Weiss!!!! Are you ever gonna block a shot? No, then don't jump for that." Maybe two games later we are versing a rival school. Kid on the other team who used to play for Jericho's travel team comes down the court on a fast break. I get to the middle of the paint and he goes right at me—I block his shot right back in his face and everyone goes nuts. It was super clean, but of course the ref blows the whistle for a foul. After the game I go up to Coach and say, "Remember how you said I would never block a shot?" And his response was, "I recall the ref saying foul." I definitely put in work defensively that season and my game's intensity developed.

Going into my junior year of high school, I felt confident that I belonged on the varsity team and wanted to show it in the preseason. Our school team entered into the preseason league and I really showed off my shooting ability and my ability to score in these games. I hit a lot of 3 pointers and put in work offensively and went all in on my defense.

Fight Through It

After the tryouts, I finally made the varsity team to play for the coach who scoffed at my wanting to play college basketball. I made the team over more than about half of the A team kids who made the team ahead of me years before, which just goes to show you that it doesn't matter where you start, but rather how you finish. This was a huge accomplishment. Then, the season started. I would get chewed out for every mistake in practice. In addition, having some teammates whom I didn't really gel with didn't make matters better. I was losing confidence at times and was very anxious. I hated going to practice, which I guess became a theme amongst all my teams. I didn't have many friends on the teams, and I often didn't feel much support from the coaches. It was often a lonely experience and it wasn't easy walking on eggshells. I just couldn't take being blamed by teammates for every mistake. I thought my teammates were supposed to support me. They displayed all this negativity towards me in this sport that I loved and worked harder to achieve in than anyone. I was always the one taking the blame and the yelling, but never dishing it out because that's just not who I am. Continually being blamed for every shot you take, every shot you miss, and for every time the other team scores on you, gets to you after a while. I felt like I became a scapegoat for everything that went wrong due to the fact that I was so nice and wasn't going to fight back. I lost a lot of confidence during this time. However, at the first scrimmage of the year a bunch of players were suspended for fooling around during our concussion test. So, I was the first point guard off the bench. Knowing that there was no one behind me, I knew I had the green light. In a couple minutes I had 2 or 3 3 pointers and 2 foul shots for either 8 or 11 points as well as 3 assists. One would've thought this would be enough to earn some playing time. For the rest of the season I didn't play much at all, until one of the later games where I came in for a couple minutes and went 2/2 shooting and had an assist. Still, even when I brought up to the coach that I think I could help the team by playing more, he said, "You're doing great in the role that you're in-you just have to keep learning and next year you'll be ready." We had a loaded senior class that year and made it all the way to the Long Island finals where we lost in a close game. It didn't really matter much to me. Yes it was cool to be a part of that team. Call me selfish but if I work harder than everyone else and I'm not able to contribute to the team product in games, I'm really not interested much in whether we win or lose, especially when the environment I was in often seemed very hostile. It's not that I didn't want to support my team. If you know me and how I treat my friends you would understand I love supporting good positive people. I was just really upset at the fact that I didn't feel the love in return from my teammates. Also, not getting my own opportunity that I worked so hard for left me bitter and upset. I often felt more in competition with them (maybe this is just how the high school sports environment is), and so I found myself feeling defensive against my own teammates and it wasn't a good feeling. After one of our big games that year Coach comes up to me and one other kid and says, "This is your team next year. We'll be back at this same place led by you guys." This gave me hope for next year.

Basketball-Preseason Senior Year

The preseason going into my senior year, my dad advised me to organize the team. As uncomfortable as it made me, I called the coach and told him what I wanted to do. My dad said this would show initiative and help me become a captain and hopefully get that star role that I worked so hard to achieve. In these games I really showed out, putting up big numbers, running a fast paced offense and even hitting a few game tying buzzer beater shots, as I was accustomed to taking throughout my career.

Then, there was a tryout to make the top 40 of Nassau County. You would be placed on a team and scrimmage for about 3 days, trying to show that you were a top 40 player against a few hundred other players who were trying out. Next, you needed at least 3 coaches from the county to vote for you to get put in the big game. I gave it my all. I felt that my tryout truly showcased my skills. The following night, I get a call from my high school varsity coach telling me that I made the team as 4 coaches voted for me, and he told me how great of an achievement this was. I was so happy and proud of myself. Then, came the Nassau vs Suffolk County game. The first play when I go in, I'm guarding a kid who many considered to be the top player on Long Island, and I decided I was gonna show no fear and guard him full court. First play he tries to cross me up, I pick his pocket (steal the ball), and miss the layup, but after that I earned a lot of people's respect. Nothing was given to me easily. My coach on that team pulls me aside after I came out the first time and says to me, "you just picked the pocket of the top guard on the whole Island, how does it feel?" My high school coach also called me afterwards to tell me he was proud of how I held my own.

My senior season rolls around. My ankles had started getting really weak from the summer before and this was the start of my ankle sprains. Whether it was the overtraining and overworking of my body without sleep, or lack of ankle mobility, or trying to brace the symptoms without addressing the source of the issue, or even nutritional deficiencies or emotional traumas (as I'll get into later on), and constantly trying to wear more protective shoes, I was constantly spraining my ankles. During the soccer season that year (before basketball season) I had started with two sprains, and the summer before I had had a pretty bad one too. Even so, basketball season started off with high expectations. I thought this is where it all pays off. I'm gonna get the recognition I deserve and get those college offers (and dunk soon too). I sprained my ankle in one of the first practices. When I came back, I was told to practice with the white team which was usually the reserves. I thought it was just temporary, until coach came up to me and said I was going to be the 6th man to start this year but I was still going to have a huge role. Major shock and disappointment. This was supposed to be my team and my year. Then one day at practice Coach starts calling me a new name, "D1." He would say it in a mocking way. I came home really upset. He came into practice the next day with sort of a backhanded apology or at least that was how I saw it. He said, "When you were in 9th grade, your dad said to me that you were gonna be a D1 player. So I told him that I would know if you were a D1 player." I begrudgingly accepted his apology even though that fire was burning in me like crazy to prove him and everyone else wrong.

It continued to become clear to me that my skills were underestimated, so while I became cynical and still hated going to the practices as I said earlier (due to the negative environment and my lack of support and recognition), I did always put forth my best effort in practices and the game. However, now looking back, I realize that maybe I was giving other people's thoughts and opinions of me too much of my energy and this brought about some negative energy from me. Maybe I was unintentionally outsourcing too much of my power to others. But at that point, that fire was burning in me like crazy to prove them and everyone else wrong. Anything was possible and I was going to show them!

The first game comes and I was pretty hyped up. I come into the game about 3-4 minutes into the 1st quarter. I catch the ball on the wing and immediately drive to the hoop and go baseline trying to lay it in with my right hand, but someone on the other team took up the space in front of me, so this should've been a blocking foul, but no call. Then the next possession I get the ball trapped in the corner during our press break and I try to dribble through it, so I get the ball stolen and Coach takes me out. I didn't come back in for the rest of that game. I was ready to quit. My dad stopped me right there and asked what I really wanted out of basketball. In other words, what comes next after high school? I said I didn't care what my stats were or anything like that—I was going to work on becoming the best player I could possibly be, and I was going to dunk soon and try to play college and maybe even pro ball. I said I just needed time. My dad said if that's what you believe then I believe in you too, and go after that with all you can. Become the best athlete you can be and you will dunk and play ball beyond high school. But, my dad said to me if you quit that would be worse, so just don't quit and keep giving it your all. I agreed that was fair. I bit the bullet. This was also one of my first realizations that working hard is amazing but it doesn't guarantee anything. You can do everything right, but you can't control others and can only control so much of your own stuff. Sometimes it's an accomplishment just to stay in the game.

The next day in school one kid was talking to me about the game last night, and I said how pissed I was at the coach for taking me out. He tells me that I should be happy that I'm even on the team because he got cut. So, I said, "Yeah but I worked super hard for this." He did have a point in that it was an accomplishment to even make the team, but he didn't get my mindset. I don't want to settle for less than I'm worth. I always want more for myself. I know I'm an underdog and don't have the size of a "typical athlete" or the natural abilities, but I have what can't be taught: the heart to go along with an insane work ethic, and I'll take that any day. The rest of that season, I played well when given the opportunity and was very efficient on offense and was a lockdown defender. Despite the coach leaving me in for brief stints, I did play in every game, one of the only players to do that. But, I wasn't given the time or the chances to put up the large numbers that I knew I was capable of. Also, one of the hardest things as an athlete is playing for a coach who takes you out after every mistake. You become afraid to take chances and to show your true potential and I played for a lot of these coaches during my high school career. The coach either didn't believe in me enough to give me more time or was holding my high belief in myself against me. Maybe he saw my large goals as selfish. I was essentially the 6th man, but I never started a game that whole year and probably didn't play more than 10-12 minutes in a single game. Not even on senior night, which was my best game of the season. Our team didn't perform the way we should have that year. We had no team chemistry and a lot of talking behind people's backs. In my opinion, none of us were played to our strengths. Going into the last game, it was senior night with our record at something like 3-16. I was really bitter about how the season went. It wasn't that it was all bad, I had accomplishments and played well when I got the chance, but it just wasn't what I had expected. Coach had 399 career wins coming into the game and was looking for number 400. One kid on the opposing team was destroying us. I came into the game and was charged with the task of guarding the kid. He had about 14 points already when I came in towards the end of the 1st quarter, and by the end of the game he finished with 18. Only two of those points were on me. I shut him down with full court defense and drained a few threes and a couple free throws of my own, and we got the win against a top team from our conference. Immediately after our game (as he had also told me in private the day before) when we were talking as a team, the coach apologized to me in front of the whole team and said, "I really am sorry that I didn't give Weiss the amount of playing time he really deserved this year. He was one of the best players on this team and I was wrong for not seeing that." It was a very nice apology and I appreciated his acknowledgement, yet I wished he would've realized it sooner.

Shortly after I got out of the hospital as I'll get to in a bit, Coach actually came over to my house to visit me. I definitely appreciated that very much, as well as all the people who came to see me and tried to lift me up when I was at my lowest. He sometimes comments on my Facebook posts to root me on in my endeavors and with especially thoughtful sentiments. As I've learned, forgiveness is for yourself. You don't have to forget or ignore what happened, but if you can't forgive, then you can't move past it and heal from whatever you felt. There is nothing wrong with feeling wronged, but it is essential to let go of the hate and anger and negative emotions that you felt, and find the good from that situation. It's also important to look back and understand that maybe there was a reason why things didn't go the way you had planned in that moment. God's plans were bigger than your own and even though you may have been tested, you were also being prepared for something much greater. I can take the good out of that situation and put a positive spin on it and move forward in a positive direction. I know that this situation doesn't even compare to any of my other challenges that I've faced since and really wasn't all bad, but it definitely inspired me to keep going and to help others with their goals and to show them that no matter what happens, you can achieve anything as long as you believe in yourself. And even after I got out of the hospital, one of the things that kept me working on myself and my game was that I knew I had to become the best player I could so I could show myself that I wasn't done yet! Another piece of forgiveness is forgiving yourself for times when you may have acted poorly or gotten upset at someone because you can't fault yourself for feeling that way, and in order for you to heal, you must also forgive whatever wrongs you may have done. The same goes for my soccer coach as well—as you will read about that whole story in a bit. Shortly after I came home from the hospital and was back on my feet, he invited me to soccer workouts with his team. This was important in regaining my confidence through movement and getting back to myself through skills and fun. I really appreciated him for inviting me to be a part of his team's workouts during this time. So the same thing with forgiveness and being able to move on and look back and understand why things didn't work out the way you had hoped, applies here.

Sports aren't always "fair," but then again life rarely is. Many things in life are out of our control, so we must control what we can: our work ethic, showing up every day and putting in 110%, and putting in the work when no one is watching. Eventually, it will pay off in some way, but as I said nothing is guaranteed. Without all of the struggles and obstacles I overcame, I wouldn't be who I am today. Also as I've learned along my spiritual journey, the joy and the reward is often in the playing and in the journey. So, there is more to it than just "winning" or "being seen as the best," as I used to think.

Jared Weiss

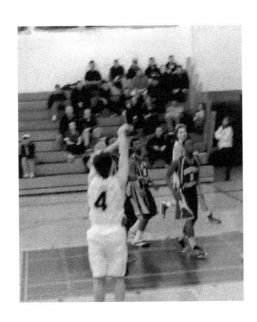

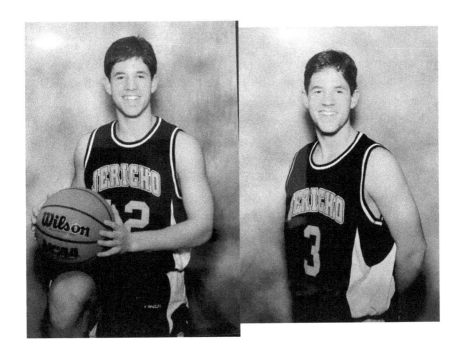

DIFFERENT STROKES FOR DIFFERENT FOLKS

Chapter 12

While I wish I could say that I always played amazing whenever I got the opportunity and that I was playing in every game in AAU, this wasn't always the case. There were plenty of games where I would have to watch the whole game from the sidelines. There were also plenty of times throughout all of my teams where my anxiety would get the best of me, as I would hear all the outside noise from everyone seemingly screaming at me, that I would become so ridden with fear and would make the wrong decision and get taken out right away. I always knew what I was capable of, but sometimes anxiety and worrying about what others thought of me would take over. There were even times where it felt so bad that I would actually start shaking or would be so afraid to shoot or do anything. This anxiety has also been one of the reasons why the hardest shot for me has always been an overhand layup. When you are expected to make the shot and know you will get yelled at if you miss, you tend to overthink it and lose the touch. I was always a better three point shooter than a layup shooter, which theoretically shouldn't make sense, but the mind can play tricks on you. Interestingly enough, when I've spoken about all of my performance anxiety with Brandon in recent years, I discovered that he actually took things in a completely opposite direction. We both played for a lot of the same teams and had the same dad coaching us on the sidelines—but I internalized everything and every time my dad was vocal with me, it hurt my ego and harbored difficult emotions. However, Brandon really didn't feel the same pressure. He had the ability to focus on the game and let it all roll off his back, as well as take it as constructive criticism. I think also he was able to not take the game SO SERIOUSLY. I guess this also goes back to how I was saying we all need individualized coaching, and you have to know your personnel, because what works for one player won't work for another. We also didn't have the same circumstances, personalities, opportunities or surroundings, such as type of friends, or the same life overall of course, so there are a lot of factors that account for this—but I found this to be super interesting. He seemed to be able to have more fun on the court, whereas for me sometimes depending on the team I was on, I was able to have fun, but other times it was like I was going into a boxing match without any headgear.

This aspect of sports was very hard on me, and when it came to healing from my major health issues later on, I realized there were other aspects of my life that could use some healing and love as well.

TRYING TO TUNE OUT THE NOISE
Chapter 13

When it came to the amount of practice I put into my game, there was no one who could compare. No one was working nearly as hard as me or putting in the reps that I was. Before practices on weekends, my dad and I would get to the gym early and put shots up. Then, one day one of my high school coaches comes up to me and says he doesn't want me practicing outside of our practices because it takes away from what we're doing as a team. Imagine that...being told I shouldn't practice? I don't know what the reasoning was, but whatever the reason, I took it personally.

You have to learn to ignore the noise and play your game. It wasn't always easy but whenever I was able to tune out the noise, my game would really take off! My dad used to encourage me all the time to shoot more, and I would become hesitant. I wasn't sure what I was supposed to do. Was I supposed to pass it to my teammates who were calling for the ball? Was I supposed to run the play that the coach wanted me to? Or was I supposed to shoot the ball? It's confusing and very anxiety provoking when you have so much outside noise telling you what to do. But, as with everything else, sometimes you have to tune out the outside noise and do what you know is best. And that truly is a big part of the game of basketball. So, if that means taking away shots from others because you know that's the right decision, then you ride with that and shoot the ball. That's also where having the right coach comes in. And as with any fear, the more times you acknowledge it, yet do the thing you want to do anyway, the more normal it will become, and you will start to gain confidence in knowing that you can do it. There were times when this got me into trouble with coaches and teammates who didn't have my best interests. Even recently, former coaches have asked me why I love scoring and shooting so much, and they asked if my dad instilled that in me, and most certainly he did. But what they don't realize is that if he hadn't, I might have remained afraid to shoot (or did he make me hesitate more, unintentionally? We'll never know...) and wouldn't have maximized my full talent. In order to be the best you, this does require working on yourself, and that doesn't make you selfish. It's looking out for your own best interests. In later years, the more I exercised my mind power and became better at dealing with my thoughts and emotions, the better my game became. Even more, this translated to all aspects of my life as I was able to block out the outside noise. What I've also learned, as I will get into a bit more later, our environments we're in will always play a role in our success no matter what we are doing. And some environments, no matter how hard we try, just aren't right for us to succeed and we may need to revamp our surroundings.

Basketball-College Camps

Towards the end of high school I attended a few college basketball camps. This was my way of betting on myself. You don't get anywhere by listening to those who tell you what you can't do and believing them, so I was gonna bet on myself and it paid off. I needed that type of "delusional" self-belief that Will Smith spoke about in these motivational videos I used to watch, where I saw what no one else saw in me and what I was capable of. The first camp I attended was at Columbia University. Let's just say the coach knew who he wanted on his team going into the camp, so he loaded up one team of players who he was really looking at and basically took everyone else's money. One day, the head coach comes in saying that he was so impressed with all these kids who had come in early to workout. The reason for this was that he told those kids who he was focusing on to come in early to make them look good. Unreal. But this is the type of politics (i.e. who you know) that happens almost everywhere in life unfortunately. That camp was a sour experience, but it didn't slow me down. A few months later I was invited to the Harvard basketball camp. And this was a totally different experience. The teams were more evenly balanced, and the competition was really tough as well. My teammates and coach happened to be really nice at this camp too, and as I've come to realize, this makes a tremendous difference when it comes to anything that you do in life. Confidence and team chemistry are everything, so having others who believe in you will inspire you to play better. Having others encourage you to show your skills and to keep shooting when you miss helps a lot. In spite of us being an undersized team, we really performed great during the games. I think the coach was still a bit skeptical of me being a legit ballplayer at first since I was the smallest on the team…until the playoffs came. The one thing you can't judge on a player or a person is how much heart they have and how much passion they play with. Stats, accolades, those things are cool—but they don't tell you about the player who has no quit in him and won't give up. Those attributes can't be measured, and those are some of the most important ones to have. Going into the first playoff game, our point guard got hurt. (I was playing some shooting guard and some point guard, but wasn't starting in these games. I was coming off the bench and playing really well with the second unit.) So, my coach (Brandon Ball), who was a former undersized hooper himself and now a college coach, tells me I'm going to be starting. I took on the challenge. The other team's point guard was arguably seen as the top player in the camp up to this point, averaging around 25 points per game and just destroying everyone. I guarded him full court and he ended the game with 6 points, and I had at least 5-6 steals and a few blocks. This kid was so frustrated he couldn't hit a shot over me that he just kept jacking them up with me draped all over him. I also chipped in with 9 points of my own and pushed the pace, ran the offense as the point guard, and we won the game in a huge surprise. After every playoff game, the coach had to choose an MVP from the winning team to show the college coaches attending the camp. My coach chose me. This was a tremendous honor. Coming to a D1 camp as a 5'6 kid who no one would've given a second thought to, and I won MVP of a playoff game. Heart over height. I'll take that every time. Little did I know that a scout from MIT was in attendance, and after the game he came up to me and my dad to tell us how impressed he was with my game and wanted me to come to MIT for a visit. My first college look was here! In the second game of the playoffs which was on the same day, I literally had no legs or energy left so the game didn't go as well, but I had proven a lot to myself. Unfortunately, I didn't get chosen to the all star game which would've probably given me a lot more looks, but I had done what nobody said I could—I believed in myself enough, and that was an amazing feeling.

I got two more college offers/looks coming from AAU tournaments (outside of school ball). The first one came prior to my 12th grade year.

One day, the athletic director, who a few years prior had doubted it was possible for me to be a college player, tells my dad that the coach from SUNY New Paltz had called his office to tell him that they were interested in me. Then post high school senior season AAU, I played really well in a couple of tournaments, including winning MVP in one while playing for Coach Ritchie. I also played for Coach Barry, as well as played for my dad and Coach Warren in tournaments in Rhode Island and Massachusetts. After one of these tournaments I started getting weekly emails from Norwich University, a military school in Vermont that really wanted me, telling me they wanted me to play for them. The MIT offer was my top choice, but first I had to get into the school. Unfortunately, this didn't end up happening. This felt like a big rejection especially because I wasn't going to take the other offers, as those schools didn't line up with my academic goals. I decided I was going to try to walk on to the team at Cornell. I thought to myself I would be the perfect walk on, I'm the hardest worker and the underdog, and I felt like that's what these coaches would love to have seen. At the time my athleticism and skills weren't what they are right now, so I most likely would have had to start on the practice squad and attempt to work my way up. I would've done anything to get on that team because I had the stuff that can't be taught: a lot of heart and a ridiculous work ethic and someone who never gives up. I was going to work my butt off to be as ready as ever for a tryout.

Soccer-High School

Towards the end of middle school and through the beginning of high school, I decided to join a camp friend of mine and take his suggestion to try out for his town's soccer A team. Along with a couple other kids from my town, I went to the tryouts and we made the team. I would play for them for 3 years and I loved it. We were starting in a fairly low division, but over the next few years we would climb up the ladder by finishing 1st in our division numerous times. Next came the tournaments. This was where my clutch genes would be revealed. In league games you didn't have shootouts, games could end in ties. But in a tournament anything goes. Two straight years we were in the Waldbaums Cup, and both years every game went into a shootout leading up to the final round, and I never lost a shootout during that time. I gained confidence and you'd see me showing off this confidence during these shootouts by doing all these mind tricks with the shooters. I saved a ton of PKs and led our team to winning the cup two years in a row. As nerve-racking as these were, I loved them. Something about the thrill was invigorating. My parents along with every other parent would be so nervous and would tell me I gave them heart attacks through all of the close calls. The whole crowd would hold their breath and tell me to try to not let the game go into a shootout. I absolutely loved the feeling when a shootout ended and my whole team would run up to me and mob me, knowing that I conquered this accomplishment and put the team on my back.

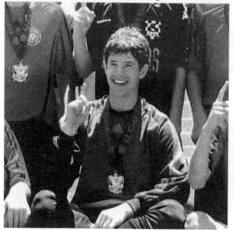
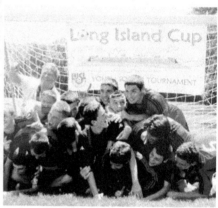

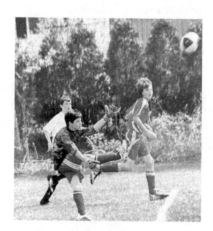

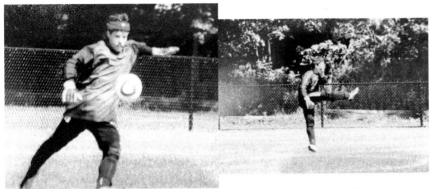

Meanwhile, when it came to the JV school team in 10th grade, the other goalie and I would split time as we would each play half the game and we had a lot of combined shutouts. In 11th grade I had to make the difficult decision to leave Syosset and play for my own town's team. The coach of Jericho's travel A team was also the coach of Jericho High School's Varsity team. Needless to say it was imperative for me to do my best to get into this coach's good graces. I also needed to learn a new position since goalie was taken by the kid with whom I split time on JV. My general athletic skills allowed me to switch off between forward, midfield, and even a bit of defense. I had played goalie all these years so it was a tough adjustment to make on the fly. There were many new abilities to master. Until one day, I find out that the goalie broke his arm and I was being asked to play goalie. I was very excited. This was also one of the first games of a tournament. And of course during that game I saved a PK and then the game went into a shootout where I made 3 saves.

Unfortunately, in 11th grade it was predetermined that the varsity team already had their two goalies selected, so I tried out as a forward. I was disappointed but there was nothing I could do about it. During the tryouts, we ran on the track and no one could keep up with me. The coach really liked this as he was a fitness buff himself. I clearly demonstrated that I wanted it more than anyone else, and I think he could see this as he was constantly complimenting my speed and the shape I was in, as well as my work ethic. But when it came to the final roster, the kids who made it were the kids with whom he worked all these years. But truthfully, this went how I expected. After all, I had been playing for another town the past 3 years—I was an outsider. I was stuck playing JV again. Even though I knew coming in that I was placed at a disadvantage, I was still really upset. The other kids were throwing up during tryouts and couldn't handle the running or the fitness. However, I had only had very limited experience playing a position other than goalie, so I was at a disadvantage. I could only control my effort and work leading up to the tryout. More doubters, more motivation, I had to keep grinding. On JV that year I would be playing forward, so I took this as a chance to work on necessary skills and to show everyone that I was good enough to make and play on varsity. First scrimmage I have a goal and an assist. Then, the second game, the coach doesn't start me. No explanation. Now, I hate confrontation, but my parents also always taught me to stand up for myself. I knew I didn't deserve this. Maybe this wasn't the right time but I didn't care. I walk up to the coach and say to him, "Why am I not starting?" He immediately got angry at me and said, "This isn't the time, go sit on the bench." I was furious, but as soon as I came in I started making things happen and had some really great crosses and even an assist or two. Over the course of that season I was 2nd on the team in goals and 1st in assists. The coach still didn't move me up to varsity for the playoffs.

Then, senior year, same type of tryout. Even though I had only made the switch from goalie to forward the year before, I had proven myself and finally made the varsity team which was a great accomplishment. I worked my butt off in practice in spite of two sprained ankles that occurred at the start of the season. It wasn't easy playing through those injuries but the coaches liked my work ethic. I made a great connection with one other kid on the reserves. We were constantly working in practice to outrun the starters and scored a lot of goals. Unfortunately the coach had already decided his lineup. I could only control how hard I worked, but I couldn't control the decision making. As usual, I tried making the most of every minute I got and hustled like crazy, trying to do all the little things. We ended up tying in the state finals so we won a part of the state title. I was part of it but it would've been nice to have more of a playing role. It was a cool thing to say, but me being the relentless competitor that I am, I wasn't as happy as I would've been had I been given the opportunity to really show my skills with more playing time. That's just who I am. I have never been someone who settled for less

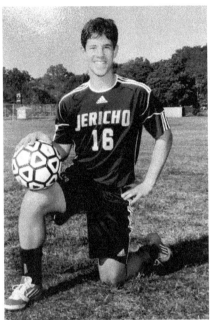

than my worth. Also, I suppose I didn't have the track record nor the opportunity to really be able to prove myself, since I had been playing goalie for another town all these years and suddenly had to learn a new position. I'm happy that I achieved making the team and being part of a state championship was an accomplishment for sure, but I still was always hungry for more success. I still needed the recognition for my hard work. Similar to how it was with basketball, it wasn't that I didn't want to root for my team, I just wished I was part of a more supportive environment with people whom I really vibed with! And more than anything, I just wanted someone to give me recognition for my effort!

Track: High School

I started running track in 9th grade as a way to get faster for basketball and soccer. I had always played baseball in the spring, but the problem was I couldn't commit to it due to my other sports. And it's really hard to not play baseball for a while and then come back and hit fastballs and curveballs. So I made the tough decision to end my baseball career (as I already mentioned). As you'll learn I have a hard time with change. I like to attempt to do it all at once and go all in, which sometimes leads to too much stress in my life, but also illustrates my desire to be the best at everything.

The first year, I was asked to be a long distance runner and I mainly ran 800m and one mile events. These didn't exactly fit my build because I was a muscular kid from all the weight training I was doing, but I also had a lot of endurance from constantly pushing myself beyond my limits. The first year went very well, and I started to treat track more as a serious sport rather than something to do on the side. I started receiving invites to the weekend invitational meets and was performing very well, especially for someone who had never run track before. I was hitting a personal best in just about every meet. The second and third years' progress stalled a bit as I was focused on basketball and soccer, and with all of that extra practice on top of my school work and weight room training, improvement was difficult. I finally broke through some plateaus and started running 400m events too. In addition, we had a sprint medley team that was very close to qualifying for nationals. I also ran for the 4x800 team. We were getting pretty good too. We were running in the counties and placing high in our conference meets. By senior year I had mostly stopped running distance and transitioned to more sprinting with 100m and 200m events to better fit my build. Something that really hurt my ego though was when my new coach took me off the 4x800 team senior year, even though my time was within a second of the kid who replaced me. It was so confusing since the coach was often commending my work ethic and I had been part of that group since freshman year. Also to not be named captain, even though I felt I deserved it, just as with basketball, was another blow to me. It was always tough not getting the recognition I felt I had earned, but this would also cultivate a mental toughness in me that I needed years later when it came to becoming a content creator.

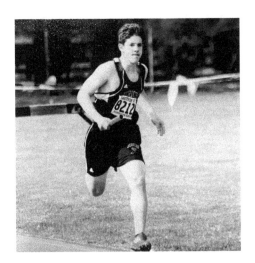 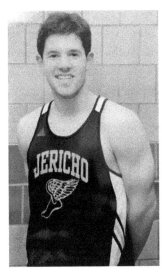

Soccer-Applying to College

When I was applying to colleges I didn't limit myself at all. I was trying out for basketball, soccer, and track. I didn't want to look back and regret not pursuing every sport. I did get one college look for soccer after sending out a bunch of tapes, and was invited to a camp at Williams College where I tried playing both goalie and a bit of defense. But, I 100% believe that had I been given more opportunities with soccer and had I focused more exclusively on it, I could've gone even further. That's always going to be my mindset, that with time and effort anything is possible for me!

For the Love of the Game or To Please Others?

I feel like a lot of times throughout my athletic career, I got so caught up in trying to seek others' approval, whether it be my dad's, my coach's or my teammates', that I wasn't playing for the joy of the game anymore. This was playing to satisfy the ego and trying to please everyone. I put a lot of pressure on myself to succeed and sometimes this grew out of control. It's a tough place to be in because I love sports, but sometimes, it just felt like I was in between a rock and a hard place and wasn't being allowed or wasn't allowing myself to just play for the love of the game.

Looking Back

I never won any individual awards with my teams in high school even though they would give out MVP, coaches award, and most improved award. At the very least, receiving the "coaches award" would've recognized my dedication to my craft and made my efforts feel validated. I was inclined to take my own path and grind in silence, so I guess the coaches didn't like my individuality. The reason I'm mentioning this is to show you that nothing is guaranteed. I used to think that being the hardest worker meant that everything would always go my way. I thought I would get ALL of the awards and all of the recognition and accolades. But...if I would've quit, I never would have reached my full potential. As Tim Grover said, "winning takes you through hell, but if you quit that's where you'll stay."

STICKING TO MY PRINCIPLES
Chapter 14

I've always been someone who lived my life guided by my principles and tried my best to live up to the high standards I set for myself. That's why it was always (and has continued to be) easy for me to say no to drugs and alcohol. Truthfully, I never even considered doing those things. That whole lifestyle of getting drunk and smoking and partying all the time never appealed to me. It wasn't in my best interests because of my commitment to health and desire to be the absolute best version of myself. In order to be the best version of yourself, it's necessary to make "sacrifices" or as I like to call them "investments," so that your future self will thank you. If you are always putting short term pleasure first, you will never get anywhere. A lot of people enjoy an occasional drink and if you are old enough and are responsible about it, then it's not terribly "wrong" to do so, as long as you don't abuse it or use it as a crutch to mask your feelings, or if it takes time away from your goals. If that's what you choose to help you enjoy yourself and relax after a tough week, and you're okay with knowing the health implications and how toxic it can be to the body, yet know how to limit yourself and can make it a super small piece of your overall routine, then by all means go ahead. But, just because it might be "cool" to be abusing these things with your friends when you're young won't make it cool if you lose control and end up dealing with the consequences somewhere down the road. Remember that all it takes is one bad decision and your whole life can be altered. Just know that every decision you make has consequences and you have to be willing to live with them. If you're getting drunk or high every weekend and during the week, your mind and body will suffer and you will be taking yourself further and further away from your goals. And if your biggest goal every weekend is to see how drunk you can get, it might be time to reevaluate your priorities. I only went to one party in all of high school with the basketball team, and then after that I went to less than a handful of camp counselor parties that my friends had hosted (post high school). I never had a desire to be part of the whole "party scene." Some of the parties I went to were pretty fun at times when the other people were ones who I liked being around. But it wasn't really my cup of tea most of the time.

There were times when I definitely enjoyed myself, even though I didn't like all of the aspects of these parties. The parties took me out of my comfort zone which can be a beneficial thing. But, I always preferred more intimate connections with people beyond just surface level conversations. Plus, as surprising as it sounds, even when you're surrounded by all of these people, it's easy to feel alone and empty if you aren't making real connections with them. My peers often found it weird that I never drank or smoked at the handful of parties that I did go to. They didn't understand how I could have fun without external substances. Some would see it as admirable and respect me for it, but for me it was an easy decision. Although it can be hard to be the only one not doing something, know that you can say no to drugs and alcohol if you don't want to partake. Be strong enough to stand alone when that is best for you and others will often respect you for it. I'm not judging anyone's lifestyle choices but I personally didn't want to rely on ANY external substances to have a good time. I prefer to feel the highs of a great workout or after playing a great game, or being in the presence of people you love and who love you. What works for me might not work for other people. Like I said I don't want this to come across like I'm judging anyone; I just don't feel that engaging in such behaviors would be beneficial for ME, and a lot of people would be better off without them too. But with any vices you may have, make sure that you are always in control and can stop them at any time so you don't endanger your life or the lives of others.

Unfortunately so many high school and college kids out there are told that doing these things is the only way to have fun and enjoy themselves. It's like people forgot how to have genuine clean fun. Especially in the case of young kids; when they get into these harmful habits, they are often unknowingly destroying their brains, ruining their bodies, and getting into trouble which is essentially setting them up for failure. And by getting into these habits, they are unknowingly teaching themselves to bury their problems and escape from them by altering their minds rather than face them. I personally always want to do things that will benefit my body, mind, and health. I have other outlets for releasing stress that I enjoy. To each his own, and I'm all for "live and let live," as long as you aren't harming anyone. I respect everybody's personal decisions, I am just explaining my personal choice to show you that although it's not easy to see, drinking or smoking is not a necessary part of "growing up" as we've been conditioned to believe. And maybe the reason why alcohol in particular is so heavily promoted in our culture is to disconnect us from our true selves and make us less healthy and more dependent. Don't forget: there's a reason why they call alcohol "spirits." If you are not careful, it can leave you more susceptible to low vibrational entities and can weaken your connection to your higher self. There's a reason why these vices are so easily available in our society; I believe it's because a population who is getting high or drunk all the time is more suggestible and easier to control. So, why not be a true "rebel" and actually become your best, healthiest, free-thinking self? Often, kids give into peer pressure for fear of not being liked. As I said earlier, do things that are in YOUR best interests and not just because everybody else is. Nobody knows what's in your best interests except you. The goal shouldn't be to fit in and be exactly like everybody else, but rather to stand out as your own person and welcome like-minded individuals into your life who love you as you are, rather than trying to make you something you're not.

MAKING MISTAKES IS THE ONLY WAY TO LEARN... (COACHING PROPERLY)
Chapter 15

As previously mentioned, I developed an uneasiness with confrontation. I don't like yelling or fighting with others. In some ways, this impacted me in sports. I'm not a naturally assertive guy so I really didn't like demanding the ball from teammates. One issue with 5 v 5 basketball is that if you're like me, you understand that when you take a shot that means that 4 others didn't. This isn't the most successful thought process for a basketball player. Unfortunately maybe I was too passive at times and unselfish. I had to force myself to become more confident. My dad was always pushing me to demand the ball. I guess I'm just not built that way. There were times when I wished I could just disappear to avoid being yelled at. I was hard enough on myself. I even got to a point where when I was practicing by myself and shooting around, with every miss, I would get so mad and start throwing the ball and become so enraged. This was not always a healthy relationship. I'm not saying that I can't take criticism and I can't take a punch, I'm super strong minded and can and have endured a lot. It's just that I internalize criticism rather than throw it back. This was something I had to work through because I couldn't let these meaningless comments stop me from going after my goals. So, as always, I had to keep moving forward and being me and bringing myself back to the love for the game. Let the critics say what they want.

It's unfortunate to see athletes give up without reaching their full potential. I'm of the opinion that the same coaching strategies don't work for everyone. I've coached kids too, not only in sports, but as a camp counselor, and by trying to be the best role model possible. The best way to help others is to know and understand who you are working with. While some people need an extra push and perform better when a coach is hard on them, others become anxious and cannot perform. Some people like me are self-motivators; we drive ourselves so when we have too many other voices in our heads, it becomes a stressful event. Other people might need the forcefulness and high intensity. And still other people need a bit of both. But ultimately, scolding every mistake without giving constructive criticism or explaining how to fix the issue leaves the kids helpless, doesn't benefit anyone, and discourages them from trying again. And in my case, this led to plenty of emotional struggles. If a player misses a shot, it is useless to yell, "How do you miss that shot?" Of course that player wants to make the shot. Then, when they catch the ball next time, they will think, "If I shoot and miss, the coach is going to yell at me." Instead they should be given something to work on like, "Hold your follow through," or be told why they missed that shot. The best way to learn is through failure. The body needs failure in order to adapt, so by not allowing kids to comfortably fail, we are stunting their growth as people. If a coach is taking a player out of the game every time he misses a shot, he will probably stop shooting. A coach can be forceful, but in a more positive way. It's amazing to see what happens when kids are given encouragement and constructive criticism rather than anger and disappointment. They get better. Things start to click. I became a much better player when I was given constructive criticism and allowed to figure things out and learn from mistakes on my own. I play the best when I'm playing with teammates who create positive energy. I never was the loudest guy in the room. I'm more of the one who prefers to lead by example and let my work do the talking. If I'm with friends, then I'll be trash talking as a joke. I'm the worst trash talker in the world according to James and my other friends as well, because they say I'm too nice lol. But, I never liked those teammates who seem to blame others for their own flaws or those who yell at others when they mess up, because failure is a necessary part of life. You have to be willing to fail in order to succeed, and if you get yelled at every time you mess up you will stop trying. I am the type of teammate and person who will always be encouraging others, whether I'm telling others to keep shooting and the shots will fall, or I'm in the weight room helping others push through their next rep and giving them the confidence they need to succeed.

The one thing that shouldn't be tolerated is a lack of effort. That is a different story because effort is the one thing that everyone has direct control over. But, the surest way to create a hostile environment is to yell and scream and single kids out. Then what happens is when a player makes a mistake, that player will blame it on another teammate, and then no one feels comfortable, and there is no chemistry. Ultimately, my message here is telling you that it's okay to mess up. Being a coach who's a positive role model can change a kid's life forever. And to all the kids out there reading this, don't let those tough coaches get you down. It's okay to mess up, even the greats fail more than anyone. Just don't give up.

FAMOUS "FAILURES"
Chapter 16

I felt that here was a good place to add in some inspirational stories from people you may have heard of who might know a little something about being told they were not good enough and may have been seen as "failures" at one point. But the reason you know their names today is because they never gave up.

First up we have one of my favorite people to follow and listen to these days, Andy Frisella. The first three years of starting up his supplement company and business he made 0 dollars. The next 10 he made 50,000 dollars total. Then, only by keeping his persistence and staying true to his belief in what he was doing and trusting God and the universe, he is currently worth multi millions. Now, for anyone who knows me, you know that I'm not a very materialistic person. I believe there is a lot more to being successful and happy than just having money. But, based on the current setup of our society, having a certain level of money can help you make more of an impact in most cases, so there's nothing wrong with striving for wealth as long as it doesn't become an obsession and corrupt you. However, a positive value system must come first as far as I see it. It should be more about what the money allows you to do, such as having the platforms to spread good will and becoming more sovereign and able to live comfortably and less dependent. Andy's perseverance and not giving up, even when he wasn't making money, is something to be admired here—plus if you can get paid doing what you love, that is the ultimate career. As Andy often talks about, every single day, the thought of quitting popped into his head. The doubts of whether he would ever make money was always lurking, but he stuck with it and now he's an incredibly successful entrepreneur and podcaster!

Moving along, we have one of my naturopathic doctors, Victor Cozzetto. Years ago he suffered from many debilitating health issues. For years, when he started his own healing process trying to heal naturally, he didn't notice any remarkable improvements, and at times actually things would look and feel worse. But as he says now, sometimes when things feel the worst, that is when the most healing is occurring. He never gave up in spite of a lot of doubt and questioning, and finally he noticed positive signs and big improvement. Then slowly but surely, more improvements came, until he became the healthiest, most vibrant self who currently helps people all around the world, like myself, heal from all kinds of 'incurable' diseases totally naturally and holistically. The medical establishment tries to convince people that healing from these labels is not possible, but you will see the proof as you go deeper into my own story.

Next up, we have Grayson Boucher, or you might know him as streetball legend and now YouTube and Instagram sensation with millions of followers, "The Professor." I used to watch AND 1 basketball growing up. It was really exciting to see all of these streetball moves and high flying dunks and exciting action going on. There was one guy who stood out, "The Professor." This guy was one of the smallest players on the court, but he crossed everybody up and could make defenders look silly and still does that to this day, only on a much larger platform. When I searched up his story in recent years it turned out this guy didn't make his high school team until his senior year. He walked on at a community college and didn't really play legit college ball, but continued to hone his craft. He didn't let others dictate his basketball future, so he tried out for the AND 1 team and made it onto the tour out of all of the other contestants. And today he is known as a basketball legend and arguably the greatest ball handler of all time.

Going along the same lines, another famous street ball player, Patrick Robinson aka Pat Da Roc. Before 2015 I didn't know much about him until my cousin Adam, who used to work for a pro basketball team that drafted Pat, asked him to send me a video to help motivate me to get better from my illness and to wish me well. He told me the 3 most important letters he ever learned, AIP, which stands for Anything Is Possible. After reading more about him, watching videos and learning more about Pat, this guy's story was prime inspiration. Similar to me, he was never a starter for his high school basketball team, even though he felt he should've been and deserved it due to his crazy work ethic. That didn't stop him from continuing to work hard. He also always had a dream of dunking despite being one of the shortest players growing up. He always wanted to play college and pro ball in spite of what others told him he couldn't do. He tried out as a walk on at his college, but got cut. Then he tried playing pro, got cut again. But, he kept working until he seized an opportunity to play for the Harlem Globetrotters. Then, he was asked to play for the AND 1 team. He also played pro/semi pro ball for numerous other teams, and today he has multiple skills academies throughout the country and is a well known trainer. He tells the people who he works with and trains that what's most important to him is that they take his message of believing in themselves and that anything is possible with them in whatever they do.

Next up, we have one of my other current favorite podcasters and someone who has opened up my mind about so much of the truth going on in this world and the spiritual war going on, Sam Tripoli. He actually has 7 podcasts but my favorite two are Tin Foil Hat and Conspiracy Social Club. He wasn't always a huge success though. He's also a comedian and knew he had a gift for speaking. But, it took him 21 years knocking on doors and getting shut down and even getting mixed up with hardcore drugs, before finally being able to make a comfortable living, in addition to becoming sober/drug free and taking control over his health! He encourages everyone once they've found what it is they want to do to, keep going until your passion becomes your career!

Last up, we have JK Rowling, better known as the author of the "Harry Potter" series. Prior to that, there was a period of time where she was living off of government welfare. At one point she was suicidal. The idea for the first book started in 1990. In 1995, she sent her first "Harry Potter" book to publishers and was promptly rejected…by 12 different publishers. In 1997, she finally found a publisher and today over 500 million copies of "Harry Potter" books have been sold.

I can find millions of other examples but, if these stories can teach you anything, it's that no matter how many times you fail, if you believe in yourself and keep trying again and again, eventually you will find success in one form or another. And sometimes, when you think you are at your lowest, you are really just building your foundation to propel you forward.

Jared Weiss

STOP CHASING STATUS
Chapter 17

There's a trap that we often fall into. It's believing that having higher status whether it be seeing a person with more money than you, seeing a kid who's more popular than you, seeing an athlete who's playing at a higher level than you, or even just seeing someone who has more followers than you, makes them a better and a happier person or that it diminishes our own accomplishments. If you want to experience the most happiness and see yourself as a better person, it has to start now, wherever you are. A thought that I've pondered is that oftentimes, God and the universe won't give you more until you've demonstrated that you can succeed and be happy and grateful with less. When you are constantly believing that you'll be happier when you reach a particular goal or when you get to a certain point in life, you realize when you get there that you are often mistaken. The happiest people know the importance of appreciating what they have right now while still being able to strive for more to benefit their future selves. When it comes to accomplishing big things, we should not be comparing ourselves to the accomplishments of others in order to look down on our own. Maybe we had to work harder or overcome more obstacles just to get to where we are, and we have to be proud of that. We all have unique journeys that we take, but I believe we can all be the hero of our stories. Only you know how hard you had to work to get to where you are in life and what you had to go through, so don't let others take that away from you. The only person you have to prove yourself to is you. Remember that your self worth comes from you! It doesn't matter if you are worldwide famous or just doing great things that might not go viral. If you are doing your best to be the best version of yourself possible and you love yourself and surround yourself with others who love you, then that is worth all of the status in the world.

5'6, BUT I WAS GOING TO DUNK A BASKETBALL

Chapter 18

I was never one to accept limitations. In my view, the limitations I have are only temporary, and with the right work I would turn these into strengths. Probably around the first time I ever watched the movie "Space Jam," I had become fascinated with the idea of dunking a basketball. Seeing someone gracefully fly through the air and then thunderously power home a slam dunk is one of the most beautiful and incredible feats I have ever seen. Growing up I had no idea how tall I was going to be, and people were always calling me short and other names associated with that. I would watch the slam dunk contests on TV, wishing that one day I would be able to do this stuff and would even attempt these dunks on my Fisher Price hoop. I watched Nate Robinson, who was only 5'9 (short by basketball standards), win 3 dunk contests in addition to being a fearless player on the court.

But, then came the 2011 college slam dunk contest. Jacob Tucker was 5'11 and came from a small Division 3 school in Illinois. He had posted a video just to get into this contest of him throwing down some ridiculous dunks and claimed to have a 50" vertical jump. He won the contest and I was amazed and immediately thought to myself, "How do I get myself jumping like that?" Bang! It was possible, someone who had probably been doubted as much as I had was doing it, why not me? Just like how everyone thought it was impossible to break the 4 minute mile until Roger Bannister came along and refused to accept those limitations. After he broke it, numerous others followed suit. (In the years following my illness, I was actually able to contact Jacob through Facebook and he was so kind, giving me tips on training and complimenting my perseverance in fighting through my illness while still attacking my goals). I called up my trainer Omar and asked, "How do I increase my vertical jump? I want to dunk a basketball." We got to work. In the meantime, I told just about everyone in school that I was going to dunk a basketball. And let me tell you, if you are not prepared for doubters and haters on the path to greatness, then you may as well stop where you are. Whether you like it or not, people don't always want to see you do well, and they especially don't want you to do better than them. I'm not sure if anyone believed me at first outside of my parents (who at the time may have only been saying to go for it to be nice and because they love me). The majority of people laughed at me. Everyone tried to tell me I was crazy, would get into my genetics, would say no one with "your genetics" has ever done this before, and make fun of my dreams. Then they would tell their friends so that they could pile on. As I said before, I was used to this, and I never let it stop me. I think I always kind of liked it when people called me crazy; it made me feel like what I was doing was special and unique. I always liked having the "black sheep" mentality and being the outlier in my way of thinking, as you'll see becoming a theme later on.

In 12th grade even my AP science teacher, after hearing about my "ridiculous" jump dreams, pulled out a yard stick to show me how hard it would be to jump 3 feet off the ground, which I had calculated would be the distance I would need to touch the rim. I would get to there and beyond; it was just going to take a long time.

"When people tell you that you can't do something, thank them because they're showing you what you have to do."-Tim Grover

WHY YOU CAN'T GIVE UP ON YOUR DREAMS-YOU NEVER KNOW WHO'S WATCHING
Chapter 19

When I was in 9th grade, I was outside in my backyard talking with my brother Brandon about basketball and our hoop dreams, and he started talking to me about what we're gonna do when we are pros. Around this time I must have been hearing a lot of my peers chatter, telling me that I was never gonna go far with basketball. Now, as I mentioned before I have never been someone who believed in setting limits on what myself or others could accomplish, but maybe my beliefs were being tested. So, I began to respond to my brother by saying, "It's gonna be really hard..." then I stopped myself, something came over me. I realized this was my 3rd grade brother I was talking to. I was not going to influence him to give up, which is when I realized I had to keep chasing my dreams too, because I knew he was watching and listening to me. So, I immediately pivoted on what I was saying, and said, "But we are definitely going to be pro basketball players." We both smiled and I had reaffirmed in my mind that I was never going to give up on my dreams. Whenever I speak to kids from that moment on, I have no problem telling them my wildest and craziest sounding dreams. Because I want them to feel that it's okay to dream big. By me saying what I plan to do, I'm giving them permission to do the same, which is an incredible thing. I can guarantee you that if you dream big and that dream scares you (as it should), you will go 100x farther than the person who let the doubt control their mind and settled for mediocre. After that talk with my brother, it breathed new life into my dreams and gave me a new responsibility to chase after my dreams relentlessly, because I had to show Brandon and all the kids out there that the world is yours and the wildest dreams are possible.

INSPIRING THE NEXT GENERATION

Chapter 20

As I mentioned earlier, I was always a very sensitive and anxious kid. Whenever others made fun of me, rather than dishing it back out to them, I took it personally and would get really upset. I think this is also part of why I am so understanding of what others go through and why I am as kind and caring as I am. I know what it feels like. When I was in elementary school and kids would tell me I had big ears, I would go home and try to push them in. Or when kids told me I was short I would go home crying and see if there was anything I could do to get taller. It was sad though because I always thought of myself as the nicest kid, yet I would get made fun of for all these things. It seemed that some people had never heard the golden rule: "Treat others the way you want to be treated." Everyone knew that I would never say anything mean back to them, so in a weird way maybe this opened me up more and made me more vulnerable. It sucks feeling like you aren't enough or that you can't do something, especially as a kid. I loved who I was, so why couldn't others see that? As time went on, I started to realize that I liked me and that was all that mattered. And then I began to attract the right people into my life. I truly believe that everything you go through in life plays into the person you become, so this transformed me into the best version of myself. Getting made fun of for being short drove me to outwork those who had the physical advantages. I set goals to become faster, stronger, and jump higher to overcome these perceived limitations. Recently when I was talking to James (whom you will meet shortly in this book) and his little brother Evan, I was telling them the importance of heart over height and saying that it doesn't matter how tall you are and to not let that stop you from accomplishing anything. I told them not to let others decide what they can and can't accomplish based on their size. They truly bought into the message. Then, Evan says, "I wouldn't mind being Jared's height. That would be awesome." By the way, I had also jumped over him (while he was standing up) 2 years prior, so I had shown him that anything is possible and now he was a believer too; so this was so special to see how I had inspired him (I wouldn't recommend trying this jump without experience). It was empowering to see the influence that I could have on this young kid—to show him that labels don't define you, whether it be physical characteristics like how tall you are or how you look, or illness labels (as I'll dive more into later on)—or any label. No matter what it is, these are all meant to keep you boxed in so that you never see how amazing and how powerful you truly are. Break through these limitations and then realize they are just illusions.

Jumping over Evan…

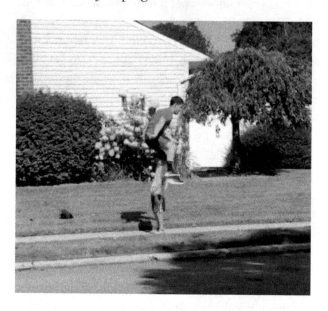

"HAPPINESS IS ONLY REAL WHEN SHARED"

Chapter 21

Throughout high school, college, and into today, I never really felt like I fit in. My way of thinking is different. The way I work is different. How I believe differently when it comes to everything going on in the world. The way I believe that I could do anything. The things I do for fun. Then, I realized why would I want to fit in when I could stand out? I have often focused on my own stuff and can be overall a very independent person. Early on there were a lot of experiences that made me feel that I didn't need others in my life… Until I found the best people and realized that everyone needs other people, and we all need to find and form our tribe, no matter how small it may be. You can get far on your own, and a lot of times you will have to walk alone when that is the best option. But the truth is, you can get much farther when you find that inner circle that enhances your life. At the end of high school in one of my classes we watched a very powerful movie called "Into The Wild." And at the end of the movie which is based on a true story, the character writes in his journal just before dying that "happiness is only real when shared." I keep a very small and tight inner circle, as I prefer to be able to give my all to each person in that circle, and I focus on quality not quantity. I have high standards for who I let into my life because I don't want to waste my time with anyone who treats me less than my best. And when you find those people who make your world a better place to live in, you never want to let them go, and you work hard to keep them happy too. Your circle will most likely change over time and it will probably shrink at times, but make sure to value those who stuck with you through it all, thick and thin. As Big Sean says in the song Too Fake, "My circle's tighter than a Cheerio."

Never let go of those who helped you get there, and try to bring them up with you. Because it is true that with others in your life, true happiness is often magnified tenfold.

LOSS AND CONFUSION
Chapter 22

Towards the end of high school, I get the news that my dad's father, my Grandpa, passed away after a long illness. He was one of the funniest people I knew, and every Friday we would see my grandparents and they always brought me and my brothers presents. My Grandma says he couldn't wait to see us every Friday as he smiled so much thinking about it. It was always so much fun talking to him about our favorite sports players and our game bets when they visited. When we heard the news that my Grandpa had passed away, it was a devastating moment to say the least. Then, not too long after that my mom's father "Mookie" got very sick and passed away. He also was one of the smartest and funniest people in the world. We would see him and Nana every week as well, usually on a Thursday, as they would always bring books for me and my brothers along with great food, and we had a ton of laughs. In high school Mookie and I would be on the phone until 4 in the morning sometimes, as he would be helping me with my AP Physics or AP Math homework. Nana would say he was so similar to me, as he was so thorough and would never give up on a problem until he finished it. When he passed away in 2014, this was yet another devastating blow to me.

Bringing this back to my own experience as you'll soon read, when I became horribly sick with my life threatening illness, my world view was shaken. I learned that life isn't always "fair." Bad things can and do happen to good people and it doesn't seem right. You can't control everything that happens to you as I once thought. Sometimes good people go through more loss and more hardship, but when you realize this is meant to or CAN strengthen you and show you your power to overcome anything, you can shift your mindset around these "bad things." As Chance Garton said when I had him on the podcast, he's discovered that oftentimes the people who go through the most challenges have the largest spiritual reservoirs. In this world there will always be duality—you can't know the amazing times without knowing what the painful or incredibly challenging times feel like. You can't know strength without knowing weakness. You always need the polarity to compare one feeling or emotion to.

Oftentimes when dealing with hardship (not loss), it is there to teach you a lesson, and then you can change your perception of these events. I believe that so much of this life is based around lessons and blessings, but you need to learn the lessons, make the necessary changes in your inner world in order for your outer world to change, because as I often say, your outer world is a reflection of your inner world much of the time.

And if you share my perspective that death isn't the end, and we are all eternal spiritual beings, this life starts to make a lot more sense, I believe (not saying that it makes losing a loved one any easier though). But, I don't see death as the end. I believe it's possible that we may even have numerous reincarnations or numerous human experiences. And with each one, maybe our soul continues to learn and grow more. Maybe there are other realms that we go into based on what we do here. But when you see us all as emanating from the same divine spirit put here to feel for God and constantly learning and serving our purpose, this starts to make some sense of these "horrible events," even though it might not make our losses feel any easier. Also, it is possible that when our loved ones pass and their human form is no longer with us, maybe they provide even more support as they watch over us as angels from the heavens. (Also, when you realize that all of us have this divine spark and that we were all made perfectly, even the worst and most painful of symptoms are there to help our bodies heal, and oftentimes we need some level of discomfort in order to grow).

Moreover, I believe in divine protection and how sometimes when things don't go your way, it's actually because God is steering you away from what isn't meant for you and guiding you back on your purpose. This may sometimes need to be a strong steer! We all experience loss and hardship but as long as you're still breathing, you still have a purpose here in this realm on this earth and can fight and heal, and that's what I want you to take away from this chapter. There were plenty of times it felt like I couldn't get through them, but I did. Nothing should stop us from rising above adversity and always striving to be the best people we can possibly be, even in the worst of circumstances.

MY AMAZING SUMMER OF 2014

Chapter 23

Going into the summer of 2014, it seemed just like any other summer, but little did I know that this would be probably the most important summer of my life. At the first camp orientation, when we found out our group assignments, I met Jacob Silverman who would be my co-counselor, and we immediately bonded over our love for fitness. I continued to meet some really awesome people, one after another. However, if there were any other signs of this being a great summer, they didn't come right away. Backtrack, one day before camp began, I had my high school graduation. Afterwards, to celebrate, my family and I went out to lunch. I ordered the whole wheat pasta with garlic and oil and broccoli and tomatoes, a seemingly innocuous and healthy dish. That night into the next morning was a nightmare. I vomited over 20 times and spent the night on the floor of the bathroom. Unfortunately I was not able to begin that summer on the right note. I missed the first day of camp. I miraculously recovered and arrived at camp for day 2 with everyone expecting me to be the savior for our group, considering the first day was a mess and they knew I had a lot of experience. What the others didn't realize is that as a counselor, I was essentially a camper. I did my job to the best of my ability, but to me that meant making sure the kids had the best time, and I wasn't going to be the guy yelling at the kids to get in line. I'm a kid in so many ways and I'm proud of it. I love to have good clean fun and make the kids as happy as possible because I know that's what I loved when I was their age. In school, kids don't always have it so easy, so I was focused on ensuring that camp would be super fun for them.

What really changed this summer though was how I learned I could have such a significant relationship and impact on a camper. Prior to this summer I always loved working with kids and had some really good groups, but something was different about this summer. I realized that this was more than just a job, but rather an experience that could honestly change my life as well as the campers' lives. Our group thrived on the balance of structure and never ending fun. One particular camper who made me realize the potential impact a counselor can have on a camper was my all time favorite camper and now my best friend, James Kass. We just hit it off right away; something in us clicked and he became my sidekick. We nicknamed him "Simba" after the Lion King. He would hold my hand whenever we walked to the next activity and on the way to all the special events. And whenever he got hurt or something bad happened, I was always the first one there to make sure he was okay, and he always did the same for me. Sitting together at lunch, and always trying to be on the same teams in sports and during our pool games would become the norm. Also, our group as a whole was just so tight knit. Some group leaders will tell their groups that "we are a family." This one actually felt like one, which is why I became so close with James as well as Jacob (co-counselor) in the years to come, and these relationships have gotten me through some of my toughest times in my life as you'll read about. From our group singing Nickelback and Aerosmith during karaoke to our group often winning the spirited competitions, and Jacob and I often having competitions to see who was more "frail," the memories will last forever. The laughs and group jokes were endless. On the last day of camp I was off to college and had to leave early. I have this burning memory of me saying goodbye to the group and the counselors and campers wishing me well, and although I am and have always been a really emotional and sensitive person, I was trying to cut it off and leave fast, as my family was waiting to drive me to school. But then as I'm walking away from 'Unicycles,' I hear James screaming, "NOOOO Jared don't leave," and he ran up to me hysterical crying, tears streaming down his face, and I got down and wrapped him up in a big hug and I started hysterical crying as well (little did we know how much our bond would only grow from there). And then the rest of the group followed. The 'Unicycle' specialist then said something that I'll never forget, **"This right here this is what it's all about. This is how you know how much of an impact you've had on every single one of their lives."** What I also realized is that this wasn't just me impacting their lives, but they impacting my life and the impression they left on me. That summer was going to be an incredible and life changing one, but not only because of what happened next, but because of the amazing bonds that were created.

DISCLAIMER: Before I go into this next chapter I wanted to make a little disclaimer. My current beliefs about what illness actually is and what causes it has changed over the past few years due to my extensive research and learning from people such as Dr. Tom Cowan, Dr. Andy Kaufman, Dr. Steph Young, Alec Zeck, Stefan Lanka, Dawn Lester and David Parker. As a result I no longer believe in many of the labels I was given, but for the sake of telling my story, I will mention what the doctors at the time told me, and later on I will go into what I believe happened. However, some things I want to get out of the way now are that I don't believe that any "viruses" have ever truly been isolated (based on plenty of experiments) and therefore are not the cause of illness; I believe what is actually being looked at are exosomes that help us adapt to our environment or just cellular debris. I don't believe bacteria or "germs" CAUSE illness either; I believe that they as well are pivotal in helping the body to clear out toxins. And just as you wouldn't blame firefighters for starting the fire just because they are at the scene when the fire is being put out, you wouldn't blame the body's mechanisms of detoxing for causing the illness. Any symptoms or responses by the body will always be healing responses. I believe that sickness is caused by toxic inputs (which I will go more in depth as to these specifically later on) that overwhelm the body, whether what you are choosing to put into your body, or environmental toxins that we don't have much control over—there are plenty of them that we are being exposed to these days—as well as malnutrition, and even emotional stressors. Also, the body never "messes up" and always has a reason for what it's doing to protect you and keep you alive, which includes producing symptoms. To be clear, I'm not saying that people don't get sick/express symptoms; the body uses this mechanism to heal and detox. And also of course this doesn't mean that what I went through was not a life threatening illness experience—IT MOST DEFINITELY WAS—as you'll read about! This will be made obvious, but I'm just claiming that the causes are not what they were initially said to be. There are many causes that I will detail in depth, but I wanted to put this out there before getting into my story.

THE FIGHT FOR MY LIFE
Chapter 24

As I mentioned at the beginning of the book, I was at Cornell and slowly getting settled in. I was doing my workout routine, practicing basketball and playing in pickup games, playing soccer with new friends, and starting my tough coursework as a nutrition major. I was meeting so many new people. This was the first time I had been away from home for an extended period of time. I had never been to sleepaway camp, and aside from the 4 day trips with my camp travel program, as well as the 3 day college recruiting camps, this was a totally new experience for me. Everything was going smoothly. I was definitely missing the incredible summer and the people who I had met and was of course missing my family. Although I was a little homesick, I had adjusted surprisingly well for someone who always got super homesick in the past when I had been away. My life seemingly felt in balance with all the pieces fitting together perfectly. My AAU coach, Torrell, suggested that I first try out for the club team as a way to let the Cornell (Varsity) coach know how I matched up against other top players at the school. Now, keep in mind that at a D1 school, there are a lot of great athletes who don't play for the main/varsity teams. So, the tryout consisted of a lot of D3 and D2 level players. When that tryout started it felt as if everything were in slow motion and it was all moving in my favor…I didn't miss a shot the whole tryout. I made 11/11 three pointers, and every time I shot the ball the other players would yell out "cash" or "money," and then splash, nothing but net. I called my parents up that night to let them know about how incredible the tryout went.

Then…BAM—it came at me like a freight train moving at full speed with nobody at the helm. On Sunday night 9/14, I had a headache. Typically no cause for concern, but my mom was worried since in the past I had had a few migraines. She told me to take Tylenol and see how I felt in the morning. The next day I woke up with a really sore throat and my energy was running on empty. But, I knew I had my second basketball tryout coming up and a lot of schoolwork to complete and didn't want to fall behind on anything. So, I got up, and while walking through the early morning darkness, pushed onward to the gym for my usual workout. I was still shooting okay but I couldn't breathe very well, and it was really hard to get through the day. I knew something was wrong but I figured it was just a cold. Upstate New York is different from Long Island since it starts to get cold sooner. But, the weather wasn't too bad yet. Me, I thought I was kinda invincible at the time. After all, I had been eating only "healthy" foods for a while now and I loved working out, never drank and never smoked, so I figured what could happen? I thought I was doing everything I could to be like a superhero. However, I didn't possess all the knowledge I have now on every aspect of health, and I didn't understand how every input affects your health, and that every element is connected. I hadn't yet learned about these things out there called toxins and where they are found, and how we are all exposed to them in various forms, and in many cases they are found in things claimed to be "healthy" for us. Also, I was so used to working myself into the ground all throughout high school and had been pushing myself and depriving myself of sleep and rest (however, I was actually making a conscious effort to get more sleep in college than I had in high school, so I had made a slight improvement there). But, at the time I thought health was essentially just about working out and eating healthy foods. I didn't see any reason why my health would be compromised in any way. As the day went on and I started feeling worse, I went to the doctor at the campus health center. I was told to put on a mask and sit in a waiting room for what felt like hours. I finally get called in and the doctor does a couple tests for strep and other illnesses. She comes back and tells me that everything came back negative, and she diagnosed me with the flu. So I go to my room to rest, while my mom was instructing me from home on what to do for my symptoms. That night I felt awful. I was throwing up a lot and not able to drink. By Tuesday morning I was completely drained. My mom told me if I felt dehydrated that I might need fluids and should go to the ER. While my mom was trying desperately to get in touch with someone on my floor who could help, she was not able to reach anyone. A friend of mine gave me the number for a taxi and I was on my way to the hospital.

I sat in triage for hours, waiting for my turn. Finally, they evaluated me and put me in a room in the ER. They set me up with IV fluids and it helped me feel better. The doctors tested for strep, spinal meningitis (scary to have a needle in your back), and other infections. While finally resting and feeling better, at around 4:00 I looked up and my mom was there. How did she get here? Looking at me in disbelief at my condition and wanting to cry, thinking about what I had been through, she couldn't believe I said, "Thanks for coming, Mom." Eyes filled with tears, she said, "You are going to be fine." The doctor came in and said that all tests came back negative for meningitis. He simply said I have the flu or a virus, and I can go home. He released me from the hospital and told me to take Tylenol and Motrin for the fever.

My mom and I stayed in a hotel where we could bring down my fever which was slowly going up. I was able to have some toast and chicken and lots of Gatorade. I remember the Yankee game on TV, even though I was throwing up through the night and spent most of the night in the bathroom. This was not new to me since I have reacted this way many times in the past when I had a bad cold, as this was my body's way of getting rid of the mucus. However, an hour by hour switch of Motrin and Tylenol as directed by the doctor seemed to do the trick. By the next morning I was feeling better. We stayed in the hotel room all day so my mom could bring me whatever I needed. She thought she was nursing the flu. I had her contact all my teachers since I was so worried about the work I had been missing. I wanted to get back to school and my routine, and mainly all I could think about was my next basketball tryout. By Thursday, I was stable and feeling better, and so my mom set me up with lots of drinks and food in my room and made arrangements to go home. But first I made sure she delivered my chemistry lab homework to my professor's class.

I rested in bed all day and later went to the dining hall to stock up. I remember talking to my brother about a new guitar he bought, and I told him I was feeling better. All was calm until the middle of the night. I felt very sick again. I dialed the phone to tell my mom. We were on the phone every half hour and she said I have to get myself to the health clinic. We were waiting until it opened in the morning.

9/19—Friday By the time morning came, I COULD NOT MOVE. All of my roommates were at classes and I was alone in my room. Luckily my cell phone was next to me. My mom called 911 to get me to the hospital. When the EMT arrived at my room, I was lying on the floor since it was cooler than my bed, but not able to move. They kept knocking on the door but I couldn't open it. They almost had to break down the door. I gathered whatever little strength I had and slowly inched my way to the door. Somehow I mustered the strength to crawl like a caterpillar and I finally got it open. They asked me lots of questions to make sure this really warranted an ambulance to the hospital (for insurance purposes). The EMTs were very nice and hooked me up to IV fluids, carried me in a stretcher to the ambulance, and we were on our way to the hospital. I was immediately placed in ICU and hooked up to IV fluids.

While my mom was traveling to get to the hospital, my dad told her that the doctor said I have pneumonia, but the reason I needed to be in ICU was only for monitoring. He also said that I was on an inhaler to get more oxygen, and in 48 hours I should start feeling better and will have a full recovery. But by the time she got to the hospital and the doctor spoke to my mom, I was on Tylenol and Motrin for a very high fever, four antibiotics since he didn't know the source of the initial infection which caused pneumonia, as well as Tamiflu in case it was the flu. He was awaiting several sputum (deep mucus for testing which was hard to get) test results. He was explaining things slowly and spoke in a quiet, concerned, and scary manner. It was good there was no fluid around the lungs which would have needed to be drained. He showed my mom the X-ray, and said I have a very severe pneumonia in both lungs and that along with antibiotics and fever reducers, respiratory therapists would need to help move the fluid along in order to expel it. When mom asked, "But he will be ok, right?" he said, "I don't know. We will do our best." My dad and Brandon arrived a few hours later.

9/20 Saturday The flu test came back negative, but they said Tamiflu can't be stopped once it is started, and there is always a chance it could be a false negative, especially due to the suspicious symptoms. We were still waiting for more viral and bacterial tests to come back. I had to take Percocet for all the pain. The next few days and nights were filled with nurses taking my temperature and all my vitals, and laying cold cloths all over me to try to reduce the fever. I had violent coughing attacks which were so beyond painful and went on for hours at a time. I was crying during them, but my mom and dad and Brandon were there with me. The football game was on TV and when I wasn't having an attack, it was good that my dad kept everything light and made jokes to try and boost my spirits, and all of ours for that matter. He was constantly speaking to the doctors and nurses to find out X-ray results and what was coming next. My dad told the doctor to tell him right away if there came a time where he was not able to treat me anymore, so that we could seek alternate medical help. Day and night the respiratory therapists (who were the nicest people according to my mom) came in every hour to turn me in my bed upside down while massaging the fluid in my lungs to move it, so it would loosen and release. Each session lasted about an hour. All through the session I coughed and coughed and coughed and coughed, while crying. My mom was always in that chair by the bed, while she watched in horror.

9/20-Later in the day...

I was in pain and so uncomfortable. My fever was going really high. They put a liquid in the drip to try to keep the mucus moist and loose. They continued with the respiratory treatments and manual therapy, but the mucus just wouldn't come up. Heart rate and blood pressure were fluctuating, and I was still on 4 antibiotics and an antiviral. The doctor was not encouraging when he spoke to my mom, but my dad said he had been speaking to the doctors all day long and that it is just taking longer than they had originally thought, but said I will recover.

I had a small window of time where I was able to eat jello, and the fever declined a little, and I was comfortable. This was one of the first weird memories I had- waking up in a hospital bed surrounded by white walls and there was jello in front of me and my mom was there and I was literally in my own world. I think this may have been right before being intubated. The doctors felt that the congestion was starting to break up. They were trying to get more sputum to test for another virus. But then the suffering started again with really scary and painful coughing episodes. The doctors said if it doesn't break up like this, they will have to do it with a tube.

The last thing I remember being asked was if it was okay for the doctors to put a tube in me, and I said yes.

The tube went down fine and they began draining the fluid. I was on a ventilator. They told us that the fluid looked better than they expected since it was not inflamed, it was frothy. They put in a bigger IV to get more nutrients into the feeding tube. All of the other tests came back negative. They were able to get a good culture and were hopeful that if they could find out what the infection is, they could better treat me. They put me on more antibiotics (21 total!) to try and cover every possible infection (*you'll soon read why I think this was absolutely crazy and could have killed me*). They expected things to move slowly. The fever started to come down. I was stable. I was comfortable. Things were finally moving in the right direction.

9/21—Sunday

Although I was sedated I was able to cough out a lot. They were continuing to clean out secretions. The doctor said we were moving in the right direction now and that I was a fighter. The secretions were not inflamed, still frothy which was good. Now they were just hoping my fever would go down more as it was fluctuating between 102 and 104. I was getting agitated and anxious while coughing and crying, but they said it was okay, and they gave me more sedatives.

They stopped some of the antibiotics, but added in different ones, hoping that one of them would work if it were bacterial pneumonia. But if it were viral, they said it just needed to run its course. Fever was finally going down. Respiratory therapists were still doing treatments all day and all night long to try and move along the stubborn sputum. Same pattern— violent episodes of coughing, stuff coming up, nebulizer, suctioning, and then sedation to manage the agitation. Fever was still fluctuating, but it was lower than it had been. My white blood cell count was down. I was stable.

9/22—Monday However, the X-ray came back not as good as the day before. Vitals were looking good, but they did have to increase my oxygen. They were still waiting for the results of 15 bacterial cultures and 5 viral cultures. If one of those would come back positive, they said they would know which antibiotic to use for treatment. In the meantime, I continued getting a little bit of so many different antibiotics as well as an antiviral.

Devastatingly, my mom and dad and Brandon had a meeting with the doctor who said, as promised, that the time had come for us to seek alternative medical care. There was nothing more the doctor could do for me here. He felt another hospital would be better as they would have more equipment to help me breathe better. He was being cautious in case I needed different treatment, and felt that now would be a good time to transfer me since my numbers and vitals were good, and I was stable. I would be transferred to Highland Hospital in Rochester under the care of Dr. Porter, the Critical Care Medical Specialist who specialized in pulmonary medicine. While everyone was crying and falling apart, I was still intubated and on a ventilator. My dad asked if he could donate his lung.

They wanted to transport me by helicopter, but it was too cloudy, so I went by ambulance from Ithaca to Rochester for a 2 hour ride that I have no recollection of. They wouldn't let my mom or dad in the ambulance, so they followed with Brandon in the car.

Upon my arrival, still heavily sedated, I went directly to ICU and was hooked up to everything imaginable. Intubated, ventilator, feeding tube, electrolyte IV, and more. They had to put a port into my chest because my arms were filled with IV lines. I even had patches on my face. However, he did remove most of the antibiotics that were unnecessary. While in the process, he asked my parents if I was ever bitten by a snake in New Mexico. When my dad said no, he promptly removed another one. Dr. Porter was confident and competent and knew exactly what to do, and he was reassuring as well. My parents felt much better. He spoke to my parents before every procedure. The main goal now was to clear my lungs and relieve inflammation. He needed to induce a medical coma as part of the treatment.

Although I was stable for a time, my fever went up really high again. The nurses would place heavy, ice cold blankets on me several times a day and night to help bring it down. The doctor said it was all a process and that we wouldn't see any results for a couple of days, until Wednesday.

While in the hospitals:

I actually didn't find out until later that I was in a coma (medically induced) for multiple days. I didn't know this until after I had come home from the hospital. As I would also discover later on, I was having hallucinations while in the coma. The reason I say I would "discover this" is because I thought these things actually happened, until I spoke about them with my mom a few months later. One involved a stuffed animal frog being on part of the feeding tube and I was holding onto him trying to save him. And also, I thought the feeding tube had these giant vegetables on it that wouldn't really go down, were hard to swallow, and were impossible to digest, so I was feeling a lot of pain during this time (my body probably was feeling pain). Then, in one hallucination I recall thinking that I had gone to one of my nurse's houses with her family for a nice dinner, even though I was sitting in a chair that I couldn't get up out of (in the hallucination). It was really shocking when I found out that these things didn't actually happen, as well as finding out that I was in a coma. I knew that what I was going through was serious, though I'm not sure at the time I even realized how serious the situation was. But I guess I was so out of it and was constantly being given these sedatives and intense medications that nothing seemed normal or real to me, just really scary. I also very vaguely remember my older brother and Brandon coming into the room to visit me. I was probably going in and out of consciousness.

9/23—Tuesday Every time Brandon or Mom and Dad came into the room, they each held my hand as I lay still. They were all terrified by my condition.

9/23—Tuesday Night Dr. Porter said that things were moving in the right direction, and we just had to be very, very patient. He said that with my resistance low from starting college and being in a new environment, I probably picked up a virus or had been exposed to some new environmental toxins in the air I had never been exposed to before. Later that night, the results came back that I tested positive for rhinovirus (a cold) and negative again for the flu. But the doctor said that there may also be another virus in the mix.

9/25—Thursday Just as the doctor had said, by Wednesday things started to improve, and he took me out of the coma. I was still intubated though, and everything else remained in place. To add more problems, during the nights I would unknowingly pull the tube out several times.

Some memories I have of this time are all of the nurses being in the room with me. I recall my mom crying and my parents being by my side this whole time.

9/28—Sunday Days and nights were extremely painful, torturous, and difficult with treatment going on. But the pneumonia was improving and things were continuing to move in the right direction. I was extubated this morning with my mom and dad right there. My mom told me she said, "best boy," and I barely whispered, "best Mom." I was speaking very softly and very slowly, and I couldn't really say too much. My throat hurt from being intubated for 10 days. My mom said I looked like I wasn't there. My eyes were glazed over. She was terrified. Of course my dad was too, but he was the rock for everybody. He always held it together.

While in Highland Hospital: Being tied down in my hospital bed was so frustrating. I had no control over my limbs. I also needed this horribly painful thing called a catheter to get me to go to the bathroom because I couldn't urinate on my own, and without going into too much detail, I'll just say it hurt a lot and was traumatizing. I also needed a bed pan considering I was unable to get up and go to the bathroom. I was just so uncomfortable in every sense of the word. Neurologists and other specialists would come see me; it was like I was a specimen being tested and wasn't human. My few saving graces were watching Fresh Prince of Bel Air at night, which my nurse Jamie happened to love too, as well as watching the Packers v Vikings game with my brother when he came to visit and the Yankee game, Derek Jeter's last one I believe. I can only imagine what others must have thought looking at me, hooked up to a million tubes, being given IV and fluids, and my whole body just looking weak. I'm gonna pause here for a second so you can get the image in your head. Then later on when you see what I'm doing now, this will be more proof to you that anything is possible.

Now, back to my hell…

9/30—Tuesday Breathing was hard, walking was impossible, going to the bathroom on my own was not even a thing. Now I was suffering terribly from medication withdrawal and post traumatic stress. My mom and dad would each try singing to me and reading books I liked as a little kid to get me to calm down and soothe me, or else the doctors would have to insert more sedatives into my tubes as my heart rate was through the roof, as was my body temperature. I had been placed in a medically induced coma for 3 days and was on a ventilator and feeding tube for 10 days. At nights I couldn't fall asleep, whether from fear of what I was going through and not knowing what was going to happen or the pain that my body was facing. I would toss and turn all night.
10/1—Wednesday But it turned out that I was suffering from much more. A neurologist came in a few times a day to assess me. Along with speech difficulties, my body was starting to have these involuntary movements, and I was hurting myself by hitting my arms on the sides of the bed. They essentially had to tie me down. My dad would try to tell the doctors that I could control these movements, but I knew I couldn't no matter how hard I tried. My brain appeared to be going haywire. The doctors told us that I was experiencing an "autoimmune" response to the infection. Interesting side note: my dad mentioned to my mom that he thought it could have been related to all of the medication and antibiotics I had been on (mostly from the first hospital). But at the time we had no clue what was causing these symptoms. In simplest terms, my body was "seemingly" attacking itself and the brain (or as I see it now, it was just reacting to all of the harmful inputs it had been given. I don't believe the body ever actually attacks itself). *(I also would find out later that the vaccine I had taken right before leaving for school likely injured me and was responsible for much*

of what I went through. I will go into more detail on this as well as my naturopaths'
beliefs on what happened in the upcoming chapters)

10/2—Thursday Dr. Porter said he thought it was the virus causing all
of this. His analysis was that my antibodies were fighting the virus, but
they also killed off some of the cells in the basal ganglia part of the brain,
which was responsible for the motor functions and soft talking.
Neurology said they could treat this with steroids or immunoglobulin, the
earlier the better. They needed to do a spinal tap yet again, a sonogram,
more blood tests, as well as sedation in order to do an MRI to check for
inflammation on the brain. So, I was still hooked up to IV fluids, 4
antibiotics, 1 antiviral (Tamiflu), continuing with the inhaler treatments,
and awaiting the results of cultures that were sent to the CDC until they
could figure out the cause. At this point, they mentioned enterovirus as a
possibility.

10/3—Friday The MRI showed no inflammation on the brain which
they said was good. Dr. Porter said the streptococcal B was responsible.
He said it typically causes bacterial pneumonia, doesn't grow in a culture,
and could result in these issues, even though this is extremely rare. I was
an interesting case for them. They did a spinal tap to search for antibodies
and the results took a while. The blood tests came back with
inflammation in my body, which meant there was a good chance I would
respond well to steroid treatment. I began steroid treatment right away. I
would then be transferred to a hospital on Long Island where they would
take over the steroid treatment, and I could be closer to home.

Dr. Porter's words to my parents:
"He is a fighter. A lot of people would not have pulled through.
He is going to live a long and healthy life.
He was put on this earth to do great things.
Lightning only strikes once."

Everything matters until you get sick, then your health is all that
matters. It took me being forced to stay in a hospital bed with these
horrifying circumstances to finally slow down. What others think of you,
or that big game, getting the job promotion, whether that person likes you
or not, how much money you make, what you got on that big test—it all
seems to matter so much until you get sick. Then when you are fighting

for your life, you realize that your health will always be the most important thing. Without that, you have nothing else. I was never used to having any down time. For me it was always go go go and if you weren't doing something you were wasting time. As much as I wish I had an endless supply of energy and capacity for work, I learned nobody does. Furthermore, being someone who always tried to be so healthy, it came as a huge shock to everyone to see me get so horribly sick. At this time, it was a mystery to all of us.

Life has a funny way of testing our belief systems. Oftentimes what you throw out into the world, the world and God will throw it right back at you to see if you're strong enough to stick to those beliefs. It's like when I say that "anything is possible" and the world says, "Try dealing with years of health issues and still go after your goals and achieve them." Or when I say, "Everything happens for a reason," the world shouts back at me by putting me in a coma and says, "find the meaning in that." Life is not easy, no one ever said it would be. But if you can turn coal into diamonds or make a great situation and find meaning through the seemingly worst of circumstances, you can achieve greatness. There will be beliefs that you will have to change or modify, just like the thought that I could control EVERYTHING. I would have to learn the long and hard way that even though you can't control EVERYTHING, you can control some things, and what you can't you have to leave up to God and the universe. And when it comes to your body, if you listen really carefully, you can hear the language of your body. Only then will you understand how much power you have. But giving up on what you don't understand never solves anything either.

It was really difficult to accept that this was my current situation. I mean let's pause for a second and recap. A few weeks prior I was a healthy college student, playing basketball and soccer at a high level, and lifting heavy weights, and now here I was fighting for my life and enduring torture. When one nurse would come, I would always throw up. Basically everything that I did was super painful. I had my parents by my bedside at all times. They are my rocks, and I don't know if I would be here today without them being there every step of the way. I was examined every day by numerous doctors. I felt like I was a pincushion with all of the needles that were going into me, and I felt like a test subject in one of those movies where the testing goes wrong and the person turns into a monster. No one had a clue what was going on with me except for Dr. Porter who knew how to treat me, as he claimed he had seen a similar thing once before, somewhat recently, with a girl who was there shortly before me.

I used to watch this motivational video where the guy would say, "When you want to succeed as bad as you want to breathe, then you'll be successful." He went on to say how most people don't know what this feels like and how when you can't breathe, the only thing you want to do is be able to breathe, and you don't think about anything else. Well, I could say I knew what it felt like to be in this position—unable to breathe on my own, unable to control my movements, unable to talk or walk— but I knew how to fight, and the one concern was staying alive. Four of the things that really kept me going at this time were 1: you could catch me practicing my basketball shooting form as best as I could from the hospital bed shortly after getting out of the coma to make sure I didn't lose that; 2: my dad would tell me all the time that he was going to buy a basketball team in Tunisia (they had recently played the US around this time) and I was gonna play pro ball for him and that I was going to be better than ever when I got out; 3: My mom would tell me every day that I was going to be okay. She would sing to me, and both she and my dad would read to me these children's books, and this was very comforting just hearing their voices, knowing that they weren't gonna let anything bad happen to me; 4: Then, the thought of getting back to camp the next summer. This fueled my recovery in a lot of ways. I couldn't let James and Jacob down, and I had to make it back to camp the next summer. This was the one thing I had to look forward to.

During this time I was forced to wear diapers and a night gown. I was coughing non stop. I was so weak, and the body that I had worked so hard to build up was withering away by the minute. This was extremely sad and almost humiliating. I was practically a baby again, and the fact that I couldn't get the words out that I wanted to say just made things that much harder. One day I couldn't poop, but I was basically told that I had to or else they would have to inject something else into me. I couldn't fathom the idea of another injection. I also couldn't fall asleep. So, my mom told me to think of a movie in my head. I pretended I was watching one of my all time favorites, "Space Jam," and it somewhat worked. I pooped and I fell asleep even if just for a really short time. I really felt bad for this one nurse because every time he came in he would have to clean up my vomit or poop. He must have really been a great man, willing to do that stuff. All of my nurses were so nice as was Dr. Porter, an angel as my parents often say.

One day after the involuntary movements had mostly stopped, I tried to get out of bed to walk with the therapist which made me pretty excited to finally get up and move. I had to hold onto a bar and the therapist wrapped this band around me so I wouldn't fall. I was in for a rude awakening. I could barely move my arms and legs. It was better than lying in bed all day as I had over the past few weeks but it wasn't the prettiest thing to see. Although the involuntary movements had mostly subsided, for some reason my wrists were curled up into this frozen position which was very painful and extremely uncomfortable. I would need my parents to turn me over at times or scratch certain parts of me, which was almost impossible due to my inability to communicate, but somehow they often figured out what I was trying to say. I was insanely frustrated.

Around 10/4 After the spinal tap came back okay, I was told that I can be transferred to a hospital closer to my home. I was free to go to hospital number 3. I was on my way in the ambulance to Cohen's Children's Hospital after saying goodbye to my lifesaving Dr. Porter and all of my fabulous nurses. The ride was to take 9 hours. With my mom right next to me, I was lying down strapped in, hooked up, and couldn't move for 9 hours. My mom sat with me while feeding me breakfast of whole wheat toast and eggs. Thank God my limbs were no longer flailing, as I had started the steroid treatment to override my *"overactive"* immune system (the quotation marks are there because my beliefs have changed and I no longer believe the body ever messes up). My wrists were still in this incredibly awkward and painful position. When I arrived I had an IV attached to me, and my older brother helped the disorganized people there get me into the bed. It was nice to have a change of scenery. Here, I was able to have more visitors come. When I first got there they would not let me eat dinner, even though I had been eating soft foods in Rochester. They said my chart showed I had swallowing difficulties. Once again, "Fall Risk" was outside my door so the nurses would know. I remember one time in the room with my mom, and I was so sad and confused about why this happened. Mom said, "It is an idiot, and it will go away" (referring to what I was going through). That made me smile. My family and some family friends stopped by, some to bring me food and also to help my mom out when she needed to leave the room for a few minutes, and some brought me sports magazines and words of encouragement. I'll never forget the people who came to visit me during this time, just as I'll never forget all those who were there for me when I needed them most in the following years. Here, I was also given my phone back, which I'm not sure how it got there or where it had been, but I guess it was unharmed. When I had a bit more control of my body I was able to look at it and see some very heartwarming texts. I couldn't look for too long because my body just didn't have the strength or energy. My uncle David came often to watch tv with me and show me videos of my cousins Amanda and Dylan wishing me well. He played a large role in my whole recovery process and is an extremely loving and caring person. My brothers were there all the time, as well as all my other family members who provided encouragement and laughs when they could. This must've been incredibly difficult for them to watch, but they put on good faces. My older brother was in college and Brandon was in middle school, so they weren't able to come every day, but when they could, they provided me the positivity that I needed. As each day went on, the pain became the slightest bit more bearable. I started taking some walks with my mom around the halls. I would sometimes tip over and fall too much one way, but my mom was there to catch me. Sleep was still very hard to come by due to the pain and the nervousness and the stress on my body, which as you'll read about would become a pattern a few years later when my ensuing health and digestive issues reached their peak. The neurologists would come in to observe me, and sometimes they would try to get me to talk which I still could not really do. I essentially spoke below a whisper and had no lung strength. In the meantime, neurologists would come in as a team of people asking me tons of questions, which I couldn't answer so my mom answered. Then this ENT doctor would come in every day saying he was told to come in to do an endoscopy to see about my swallowing issues. Every day my mom promptly sent him away, as she was very protective over me and didn't want me having another unnecessary and invasive procedure done.

It could take me up to 2 hours to eat a sandwich. My mom fed it to me in very small bites. She would feed me every meal. Getting nutrients into me during this time was crucial to my progress and helping me turn a corner. Hospital staff would understandably not have the time to stand next to me for 2 hours while I finished one meal.

After a few weeks in this hospital it was time to move on to the last hospital, which was a rehabilitation hospital in New York City, NYU Rusk. I was transported here in similar fashion, by ambulance, with my mom right next to me. When I got there, I was hoping for just a short stay and thought these people were going to heal me back to 100%. The rooms were nicer and more spread apart, and this place had a larger focus on the therapy part of it all. Just about every day I would be meeting with a speech therapist, a physical therapist, and an occupational therapist. Oftentimes the head doctor would come in the room as well to check on my progress. A psychologist came in every day too. I was further away from home as this was in the city, and after a few days here it seemed as if I would never be allowed home. My hands/wrists had felt better by this point, and I could make some sounds, just not clearly at all. I was still on tapering doses of steroids and had to avoid a lot of foods, so as to not interfere with the medication which I was now taking orally instead of through an IV. The meds tasted awful and I would put them in apple sauce, yet I almost gagged whenever I took them. It was like eating chalk. Additionally, I was given an antacid each time I took the steroids. I still was not sleeping much at all as the discomfort and anxiety was still too much. I was starting to be able to move a bit better here. My mom and I would go for walks often around the halls just as she had with my grandfather (Mookie) a few years prior when he was going through cancer treatment. My family and extended family were able to come visit more often here. I was using my phone a little bit to text a couple people and let them in on my situation, yet most of them still had no clue where I had been and the hell that I was going through. I was still coughing a lot and couldn't really swallow foods that well without coughing due to many causes, one of them being my mouth muscle strength was so weak. One day I was weighed at 110 lbs. By the end of high school I had worked my way up to around 150-155 lbs of solid muscle. My body looked so weak and bloated from the steroids/prednisone, but when I would look in the mirror I would still try to pop my pecs to show myself I could still do it. And as I mentioned back at Highland, you could catch me practicing my basketball shooting form as best as I could from the hospital bed to make

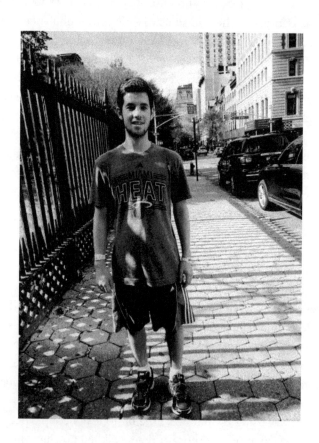

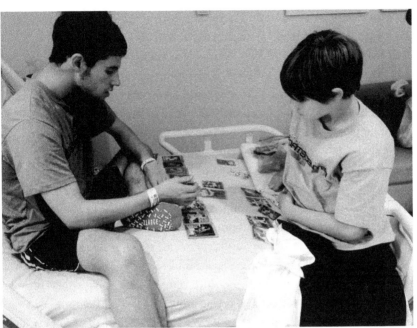

sure I didn't lose that either. My older brother came to visit me just about every day after his classes were over. Brandon visited often with my dad as well. Brandon and I played showdown cards on my bed. My mom was still staying with me as she would not leave my side. Both grandmas would spend some time with me there as well. With my nana we played cards and had dinner and watched tv, and with my grandma we had dinner and watched tv as well, and she tried asking questions to my nurses. My uncle David was still visiting often, and one night we took a karate class together (given by the hospital), which I really appreciated him doing with me. My aunt Laura and I had always joked about how we loved these Vita Top muffins. When she brought them to me, I enjoyed them so much that I felt "normal" for a few minutes. Another night my older brother and I sat in the lounge area and watched the movie *Moneyball*. He even helped me with walking to the bathroom and made sure to stand close by, since I was a fall risk. And Brandon and I would watch football games when he would come on Sundays. Everyone would try to understand what I was saying and what I wanted, as my speech was so badly slurred. Brandon was the only one who sometimes knew what I was saying; I guess we've always had an unspoken connection from all of that time we spent together. It was super frustrating. It was like I was a

115

baby with the mind of an adult. I knew that I wasn't being understood, yet I knew what I wanted to say. I started trying to feed myself a bit to get myself back to normal, but often I would lose energy and become too tired to do it, and mom would have to finish the job. In occupational therapy I would have to practice typing and doing brain games on the computer. I was still pretty good with that stuff so that part didn't take too long to get back. At physical therapy, which happened to be my favorite, I started lifting weights again, practicing walking and going up the stairs, stretching and being tested on these things. With the lifting, I could barely get up 5 lbs, and I had no dexterity or control of my limbs. I was relearning everything that used to come so naturally. At first I could barely get up 1 flight of stairs without being out of breath and out of strength. By the end I was going up 20 flights of stairs, making pretend I was Sylvester Stallone in the movie *Rocky*, and was going past my dad who was "training" with me. Some of the stuff that we were doing would make me so frustrated and I would start crying and give up until my mom or dad would convince me to keep trying over and over again. They never let me get too down on myself! I even got to walk outside to a park one day, which was really exciting to finally breathe in some fresh air and get some sunlight after not having any for 4 STRAIGHT WEEKS! One of my physical therapists was a former college soccer player and she knew I liked soccer too, so a couple times she would set up some cones and have me dribble in and out of them, as well as have me learn other soccer drills too. Then, one day she had the idea that I could go outside and play basketball. I was so excited, it felt like the first time I was ever playing. I laced up my sneakers and put on my bar mitzvah sweatshirt, which has a picture of "Air Jordan" but instead says "Air Jared" on the back of it. We walked down to the courts which were at a park about a block over from the hospital. I grab the ball, take the first shot and…airball. It was as if all of the life had been sucked out of me. I took a bunch more shots and I couldn't even reach the rim most of the time. I was so dejected and disappointed. I started balling out in tears. This wasn't where I was supposed to be. I was supposed to be having fun at college and playing

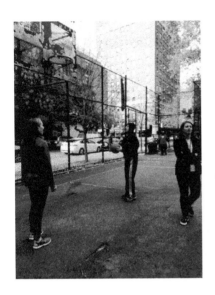
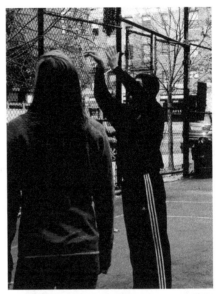
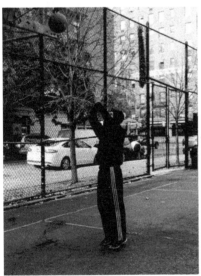
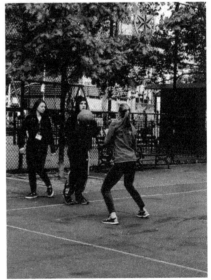

college basketball and onto my goals of dunking, and here I was unable to reach the rim on most shots. I don't know if I made one shot all day (maybe I made one?). My mom and therapist encouraged me to keep going, but after some time my therapist thought of some good footwork drills that we could do. Surprisingly I wasn't as bad at these as I thought I would be. Maybe there still was some hope. Then, my dad tried to get me back to jumping. He wanted me to feel confident that my body could do

it. The first few tries I was not getting off the floor. My body was afraid
and too weak to have me jumping. My dad thought this was all in my
head. One day a psychologist came into my room to see if I wanted to talk
about everything I had been through and see if he could help me get
through all this. It just made me more frustrated because he couldn't
understand what I was saying. My dad really wanted to see if he could
help me start jumping again. Then my physical therapist got the idea to
pull out a little trampoline to have me bounce on that, and here I was able
to get up a tiny bit. I still wasn't really able to jump on the ground but this
was a start. There was also this breathing tube/device I was supposed to
use to practice building my lung capacity, but whenever I used it I would
start getting anxious and coughing as it was too hard for me. In addition
to all of that, I was seeing a speech therapist most days. We worked on
producing sound and trying to position my tongue in the right places to
say certain words. It was difficult as was everything else, but I knew I
wanted to get better and I would do whatever it took. I would practice
with my mom in the room in between sessions. There was the tiniest bit
of improvement each day, but something is better than nothing especially
after what I had gone through. At this hospital, there was one doctor who
was in charge of when you can leave and go home, and you basically had
to impress her enough to make her think you were well enough to be
released. She would check in on me and ask me to say a few things like
my name and birthday which I could barely get out. But my release was
prevented every time I would experience involuntary tongue moving.
They said this was very dangerous. I was awake all night, every night, due
in large part to the medications, but also due to intense anxiety. My mom
and I watched reruns of The Odd Couple DVDs all through these nights.
One particular night at 3 AM, the involuntary tongue movements got so
scary that my mom called my dad who raced over to the hospital at full
speed. They told us that sometimes when steroid amounts are decreased a
bit, the movements and tremors return. When this happened, the next
day, the dose of steroids was not decreased. The doctor told us that the
"virus" may not have left yet (once again, as I'll get into later, no virus has
ever been isolated and found to be the cause of disease). Or she said it
could be transient. I really just wanted to go home already. I had been in
these hospitals for too long and was going crazy. I couldn't bear it any

longer. I felt trapped, in my head, in my body, and in this place. I really felt like I had always been so independent and self-motivated, so I thought to myself maybe I could make the most progress if I were home and working on building MYSELF back up from the bottom. I knew I could do it, I just had to be given the chance. One day towards the end of my stay, my older brother took me in the elevator and we went up to a different floor which led us outside on a terrace. It was a beautiful day and the sun felt so good. The day finally came, I was able to be released from

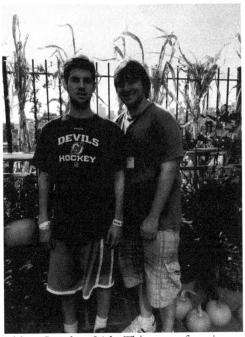

the hospital on Friday, October 24th. This part of my journey was finally coming to an end. I was still a really long way from feeling all better, but I didn't know that because my dad would tell me that within a few weeks my speech would be all better, I would be off the steroids and everything would be back to normal. I had no clue what the next several years held in store. And I certainly didn't realize all of the detrimental effects that would ensue as a result of the copious amounts of medication I was on. I arrived home a week before Brandon's bar mitzvah.

To sum things up, I had been unable to walk or talk for weeks, and then when my voice came back I would be dealing with slurred speech, possibly permanently (according to the doctors). This was my reality that I had to face. During these 6 weeks, I had been in 4 different hospitals, and over the next 6 months I'd be on tapering doses of the steroids and antacid medication. As difficult of a situation as this was, I soon learned that the next several years would be incredibly challenging, and I had a tough road ahead. I had to make the decision to be tougher than my life was. I always thought I was strong, but the truth is you don't know what your true strength is until you are fighting to keep death away and are fighting for every breath and every minute is a struggle. Severe adversity can cripple some and strengthen others. You can either give up and let your circumstances win, or you can make the decision that you have a lot more living to do, and start the fight and do whatever it takes. That's the level of grit that's required. It's okay and normal to be scared as I was, it's okay to cry a lot and let your emotions go, and it's okay to be angry at the situation in which you are placed, but it is never okay to give up. When life tests you, you've got to show it that you are a winner and no matter how bad it gets, you will not give in. This is true courage, this is what it means to overcome the obstacles and to defeat adversity. Never give up, never back down. In the coming years I'd be faced with that decision to give up a ridiculous number of times.

There was never any true diagnosis, and we were just told that there was a 1 in a million chance that this could ever happen, however I was determined to uncover the truth behind what caused this. As I've learned, I was probably better off not being given a concrete diagnosis because when you get labeled by the medical industry with this diagnosis, these labels carry weight and often preclude healing, as you will associate yourself with that condition that as some would say can't ever be healed. The body doesn't need a label to heal. But, maybe the reason the whole thing was left open ended was so that I could go on this journey and do all of my current research to figure it all out. Because the more I've gone down the rabbit hole, and the more I go through my healing journey and find these amazing people who put out incredible information on the true nature of the body, and continue with my own research, the closer I feel I've gotten to understanding what happened. Also, maybe it's also like Neo in the Matrix or Will Smith in IRobot—I was the perfect person to go through this, because it was meant for me to discover my truth and then help others. Later on in the book, you will read about my theories, which are based on 9 years of research and having spoken with some brilliant people in the natural health world.

PTSD and Psychologist

After going through the hell that I experienced, I didn't realize that I was going to have severe PTSD (post traumatic stress disorder). What this means is that I was going to have mental discomfort every time I thought of the trauma that I had experienced, and I was going to need help discussing things to get me through this. I became a hypochondriac as well. Basically every time I experienced a symptom, I would go online and find all of the possible illnesses that these symptoms are related to and then think I was going to die and immediately start freaking out. This led to multiple panic attacks and times of intense anxiety. No one could understand what was going on with me, and I felt powerless due to the thought that my body had messed up, which I would learn later on was not the case. As I have learned throughout my life, my own mind and my thoughts could sometimes be the most difficult things that I have to deal with. It also didn't help that the medication I was on was messing with my psyche and every function in my body as well, since it had numerous side effects. I began seeing some psychologists, and the first one wasn't helping much so we went to a new one. This psychologist was really good and very helpful and preached the ideas of cognitive behavioral therapy. Slowly but surely I was able to feel in control more often, rather than allow my thoughts that were running wild to control me. It also helped that I started to become a bit more active and do more things for myself, and coming off the meds helped tremendously too.

Even to this day, I still go through times of anxiety and at times depression, but I am in a much better place with my emotions and know how to navigate through these times better. In addition, I know that each of my thoughts and emotions are not necessarily bad or there to bring me down; sometimes I just have to work through them or find the lessons in them. As the famous quote goes, "You can't stop the waves but you can learn to surf." Also, having done the inner work both emotionally and physically through my holistic healing journey has put me in a much better place. Having intense emotions from time to time is totally normal, it's just a matter of not pushing them away and trying to learn from what they are trying to teach you. I am just someone who happens to be very sensitive and very in touch with my emotions, which isn't a bad thing—

it's actually awesome to be able to feel so deeply. It just means that I experience things on a deeper level; but I understand what it all means now. I also learned not to let your emotions run your whole life and influence too much of your decision making. This is where the behavioral part of the therapy comes in, listening to and feeling your emotions, but then making the best decision for you based on what you predict will produce the best outcome. Emotions and especially your gut feelings can be very useful in a lot of cases, but when you let your emotions run your whole life, you often end up in a bad place. Meditation has been one of the most incredible tools for me and it has taught me not to push my thoughts away, but to listen to them and to allow my body to experience and really feel whatever emotions I'm experiencing. This helps to allow them to pass through and then be released when my body is ready to. Attaining true inner peace is a lifelong journey. The summer of 2015 was a monumental one for me in reducing my horrible panic attacks and anxiety symptoms. Because as anyone who's dealt with anxiety for any period of time knows, being left alone with too much time for your thoughts is one of the main triggers. That summer brought me to a happy place and one that I didn't want to leave. It was super important for me to be back with the campers and counselors that summer. Having people to talk to like my best friends and family also means the world to me when it comes to dealing with my emotions. Life isn't easy but when you get to experience the amazing things, it makes it all worth it. You have to accept the totality of the experience. I am someone who goes all in on whatever I do, so I experience the highest of highs, but must accept that this also means an equal and opposite direction of lows when that experience is over. That's a part of me, and I would rather go about my life like that than only giving my half effort into what I'm doing.

Considering alternative treatment 1/4/15 due to frustration with speech

At the start of 2015, there was a potential treatment method that was suggested to me known as IVIG (Intravenous Immunoglobulin) Therapy, which was supposed to collect the "overload" of antibodies and take them away from nerve cells related to my speech issues. The doctors told me that there were no guarantees. This would have been a 3 day procedure where I'd be uncomfortable and would be injected with blood antibodies prepared from the blood donated by thousands of people. However, the day before I was supposed to get the treatment, I backed out after being told there was basically a 1 in a million chance that the treatment could give me AIDS. After what I had just been through, 1 in a million didn't mean anything to me. And truthfully, with everything I have learned since about holistic health and how the body actually goes about healing, I don't believe the treatment would have improved my condition and probably would have put me at risk for further complications. The body is never wrong as it doesn't make mistakes. There is a reason for every symptom that occurs. So the body was just reacting to harmful inputs it had been given. And there is no shortcut to "overriding it," without ultimately creating more issues. Oftentimes the path you have to take is the harder one, but is also the one that ends up being right for you, as well as more fulfilling. Too many choose the easier path that takes no effort and no work and realize that path didn't lead them to their destination. There are no shortcuts to healing, and a lot of it comes down to trusting the body and allowing it to heal at the speed it knows how to. However, there are tools and guides to help your body which should not be overlooked. I have learned that you can't fight against nature and win. In other words, you don't want to be suppressing or trying to go against the body's symptoms. Understand why your body is expressing in this way, find the root cause, and then you can aid and assist the process by helping it accomplish this task and removing what doesn't belong! It's up to you to place your body in the right environment so it can adapt and heal.

Interestingly enough, while reading *What Really Makes You Ill?* by Dawn Lester and David Parker, there was a piece that was particularly relevant to my situation. "A 2011 article entitled *Guillain-Barre Syndrome after Gardasil vaccination*: data from VAERS 2006-2009 refers to the incidence of post-Gardasil GBS (the technical medical definition is a condition occurring when your body's immune system attacks your nerves and can cause paralysis and can result in speech or motor patterns issues) as being 'higher than that of the general population.' The fact that neurotoxic substances such as aluminum, formaldehyde and mercury are ingredients of vaccines offers a more than plausible explanation for damage to nerves following the administration of certain vaccinations."

They then go on to say according to the medical establishment there are no "cures" for this condition, but they of course offer their own "treatments, which unusually are required to be administered within a hospital setting. These treatments are intravenous immunoglobulin (IVIG) and plasma exchange, both of which are firmly based on the theory that claims disease is due to a faulty immune system that attacks it's host body...the body is a self-healing organism; the perpetuation of the erroneous belief that it is capable of attacking itself, even by mistake, poses a serious obstacle to a genuine understanding of any of the debilitating conditions referred to as autoimmune diseases." As I will speak about in a bit, one of my suspicions has been that the Gardasil vaccine I received prior to college was a massive factor in my getting so sick in the first place. This assumption has been discussed at length and has since been confirmed by my healing guides/naturopaths who have looked into my case and based this on years of research, as well as patients having experienced similar reactions and symptoms. And even though I never received a definitive medical diagnosis, one of my neurologists actually diagnosed me with Guillain-Barre Syndrome on my medical report. It is also clear that my intuition was correct in not going forward with the IVIG, as this most likely would have pulled me further away from healing. The mystery continues to be unraveled.

WORKING MY WAY BACK UP FROM THE BASEMENT...LITERALLY
Chapter 25

When I finally came home from the hospital on October 24ᵗʰ, 2014, the day before my brother's birthday and a week before his bar mitzvah, I knew I was still far from better, although I was in a much more stable place. I really couldn't stand being in a hospital bed any longer, and I had faith that I could get more strength back on my own. I still had very little control over my limbs or my brain and had almost zero strength. Lifting 5 pounds was tough for me, and I lost my abs and muscles that I had worked so hard to achieve. On top of that, my vertical jump was at 0 inches. This is what rock bottom looks like from a physical standpoint. I was starting over. I really wanted to look somewhat good for the bar mitzvah even though of course that was the least of my struggles. But, so many people were going to be there who didn't know the hell I had just been through, so I didn't want to look like some out of shape college kid (not that it mattered). I started with bodyweight exercises: I started out doing push-ups on my knees and some sit-ups here and there, as well as just taking walks—it would've seemed like nothing to my old self, but in this current body it was hard. For someone with all of my athletic and fitness goals, this was so debilitating. In addition, I was attempting to do basketball workouts with Brandon, who was so supportive and always is. His patience and work with me was as he said—a way of returning the favor for all of the help I had given him. He trained me in basketball and played a huge role in getting me back to myself. I was starting from ground zero and was still on meds, so basically every bit of exercise I did was gonna wear me out.

At Brandon's bar mitzvah I managed to have a great time in spite of barely being able to move very well or speak at all. It was still mostly hand motions: thumbs up or down when I was asked a question, just as it had been in the hospital. At the time it almost felt like I was in someone else's body, plus being on the prednisone stripped my energy and gave me horrendous mood swings and made me just feel extremely out of it. I was retaining a ton of water weight, which made me upset to see where my current physique was. But, I danced the night away with the dancers who were there and had a great time, making the most of it just as I always have done. By the end of the night I left with a terrible headache and my body felt pretty bad, but I knew that I made it through, and it made Brandon happy to see me back in action. I wanted to show others and prove to myself that I was still going and had a lot more living to do. As I fell asleep in the car ride home on Brandon's lap, I was proud of myself, but knew I had a long road ahead of me.

Soon after, we started playing more basketball again, the sport that brought our whole family together and made us feel strongly connected. Those first few times were some of the most difficult ever…I could barely reach the rim on most of my shots; I had no coordination, no dribbling or jumping ability, and (this is hard to write) on more than one occasion I stormed off the court from our backyard into the house crying and cursing at my current state (which is something that I don't ever do, so this shows how angry I was). And the truth is I had every right to be upset, had every right to cry, but the one thing I couldn't do was give up. I had made it this far and I could not stop. This is where family and friends became essential. Brandon and my parents got me back on that court every time, and soon enough I was back to draining 3 pointers. Then came two of my old basketball coaches (one was also my personal trainer in HS). I got back into training a bit with Ritchie, the basketball coach who was the first one to give me the confidence to believe in myself. And of course Omar texted a few weeks after being home and wanted to see what was up. I told him everything that I had been through. That night he came to my house. He felt awful for me, knowing how hard of a worker I was in the gym, on the courts and fields, and the classroom. But one of the first things he said was, "Let's get to work." This was exactly what I needed, any form of support to help me in my quest to get back to who I was. My parents were skeptical at first, knowing the type of workouts that we used to do, but Omar assured them that we would progress slowly. At this time, every week I was getting physical, occupational, and speech therapy. I "graduated" from occupational and physical therapy rather quickly (1 month of occupational and 2.5 months of physical therapy). I stuck with the speech therapy for over 2 years though. My two speech therapists were Mara and Maggie, and both were such kind, amazing people. And even though they were not able to take me to a full recovery as the problems were deeper, and as more speech issues ensued which, compounded the situation, it definitely helped at the time to see slow progress early on due to my regaining some strength in my mouth muscles. As a result, I was much better than where I started. And most importantly, they would help me gain confidence, especially when it was time to work at camp around the kids. In addition to these therapies, Omar would come down to the basement and we got to work, starting small and slowly but surely bringing me back to my form. He was there for every step of the physical development and soon became an emotional help as well. Whenever I would have a panic attack or think I was having a heart attack or notice some weird muscle twitches or weird body pains, he would assure me that I was okay. How, you ask? By making me do 20 push-ups, 20 sit-ups, 20 burpees and showing me that I didn't die, as well as walking me through all of my fears, usually cracking some jokes at the end too. It didn't completely assure me, but while he was there I felt safe. All of this training was going on in the basement of my house and the lowest of lows emotionally. People are always talking about starting from the bottom and putting in the work when no one is watching. This was basically the definition of that. It doesn't get more unwatchable or much lower than that. I think this is one of the most admirable things that can be done, building yourself back up from the doldrums of life.

Omar came 3-4 times per week starting with basic movements and slowly trying to add weight and add more difficult exercises. He wouldn't allow me to stop when I got frustrated. And he wouldn't let me use the word "can't." We were working in the freakin basement for hours at a time. Not what I expected to be doing as an 18 year old "college" kid.

After about 6-8 months of training with Omar, I was starting to look like my old self again. Not there yet, but I was looking pretty strong, and my motor movements and coordination were back to normal. During this time, due to the steroids I was still on, I was eating ridiculous amounts of food. I was hungry all the time. Also, if you recall I had lost 40 pounds while in the hospitals. I would order in lunch daily from my favorite healthy restaurant Fuel Cafe. All the food I would get was "healthy." I wasn't on any specific diet at the time, but I was just eating massive quantities of food.

Nutrition/Fitness Interest Post Hospital Illness:

As I told you earlier, I hadn't eaten anything that I considered "unhealthy" since the 8th grade. I was in a better place when it came to eating enough, but my desire for success made me want to take things to another level. Starting while I was at Cornell, I was doing a lot of research on my own on the best diets for athletes and found a lot of good information on avoiding processed foods. At this time I adopted a diet that cut out most of my protein bars that I used to love, choosing to eat more natural proteins and only occasionally have a protein shake. I have crazy amounts of discipline if you can't already tell. If you tell me to do something and can prove that it works, I will do it 1000%. Shortly after I went through my severe illness that almost ended my life, I was looking for ways to prevent something like that from ever happening again—although at the time we still had zero clue as to why it even happened in the first place...

If any of you have ever seen the movie *Bleed for This*, the training scenes when Vinny returns from the hospital are sort of how I felt. He had been in a severe car accident, and although his situation was very different from my own, plummeting from being a high level athlete to needing help feeding yourself, as well as moving on your own and starting from rock bottom, was similar. Also, his training scenes where he's in the basement struggling to lift weights he would've easily moved in the past was relatable to my training journey as well. I had to start over again, as frustrating as that was. During my training in the basement with Omar, I had also started going back to the gym in spurts at Lifetime Fitness. I didn't do this too often because while on the steroids (prednisone), I was told that "my immunity was compromised so I really couldn't afford to get sick." During my first time back in the gym, my dad was wiping off all of the equipment which was a very funny sight if you know my dad.

FORGING AHEAD

Chapter 26

In February of 2015, one of my former high school gym teachers who I really liked texted me (as had a few teachers) upon hearing of my illness, and told me about this great fitness concept that he had just started doing called Crossfit. He knew I was into fitness because he was actually the original strength and conditioning coach during my middle school days, and he was the varsity football coach. Sometimes over the summer he would let me join in the football based conditioning workouts. He loved my work ethic. So, I did some research and it seemed right up my alley. Mr. Martinez (Will) really wanted to help me get better. I had been through a lot with Omar and had gotten to a much better place, so now I felt it was time to move on to the gyms. By the end of April 2015 I was finally in the right place to try it out. Omar had started me from the bottom and I was ready to try my hand at a new challenge. He totally supported it as he was also moving to Maine shortly after. This was the perfect timing. I also had to convince my parents that this was a good thing to do. I met with the head trainer at Light Speed Crossfit, Ryan, and attended the introductory courses where I learned a bunch of new movements and was told how a typical class worked. He could tell right away that I was dedicated and determined and a really hard worker, and he was very impressed with how I was back in the gym just months after being in a coma and going through a life threatening illness. My dad spoke with him and he approved. I started joining Will in the 5 am classes and absolutely loved it. Everyone was so supportive and encouraging. This was exactly what I needed. I was pushing my limits and moving weights in fun and explosive ways that I had never done before. My athleticism was improving at a really fast rate as well. I came into that summer with a lot more confidence than I would have otherwise. I even had an article written about my story by Ryan.

Anything is Possible
by Ryan Saraco and Jared Weiss
Ryan Saraco, Head Coach at Light Speed CrossFit in Syosset, NY, shares the inspirational story of Jared Weiss, who has used CrossFit to help overcome tragedy and turn it to triumph.

129

Fight Through It

One of our members, a physical education teacher and coach at one of the local High Schools, came up to me one morning and said that he wants to bring one of his former students in. He began telling me a little bit about his story, and I almost immediately became overwhelmed. I knew this kid was special, and while I had never heard anything quite like his story, I was excited for the opportunity to work with him. Walking into a CrossFit gym just six months after being placed into a medically induced coma takes a special kind of person.

The first thing anyone who talks about Jared says is what a great kid he is. Jared Weiss, an 18 year old college freshman, is one of the hardest working kids I've ever met. From the moment he walked in the door for foundations, I could tell he was eager to learn, to perform every movement correctly, and to outwork everyone around him. A month into CrossFit, we were doing a long workout, capped at 20 minutes. Once that 20 minute mark came around, the entire class collectively dropped to the floor to catch their breaths, and began to clean up their weights. There was one athlete who refused to finish until the workout was completed. Jared continued for another 4 minutes until he completed the full workout. It was at that moment it all made sense.

Jared is not your typical 18 year old, he's always been a perfectionist and done everything the right way. Not only did he excel in school by staying up late to finish all his school work as best he could, but he would wake up the following morning before 6am every day to train for basketball, soccer, and track. Anything to give him an edge on his competition, he would work to accomplish. He was drawn to hard work, believing that success derived by working for it is much more fulfilling than those who had it handed to them. At 5'-6", Jared had nothing handed to him, yet all his hard work earned him several Division 3 scholarship offers. The drive to prove to all those who doubted his physical abilities kept him going and excelling in Varsity sports. It also led him to turn down those offers. Jared was accepted to Cornell, and believed that along with that Ivy League education, he would be able to work hard and walk on the Varsity Basketball team. He began his first semester with the same work ethic that got him there, getting up every morning and training to get the most out of the body that genetics gave him. Only 3 weeks into his first semester, tragedy struck.

On September 14ₐ, 2014, Jared contracted pneumonia from a friend at school. It hit Jared hard, much harder than your typical case. Doctors couldn't get it under control, and to treat it they placed Jared into a medically induced coma. As he lay in a coma for two days, his body began to try and fight off the infection. This led to another unexpected result. Jared's body had a severe autoimmune response, and began not only fighting the infection, but fighting his own healthy tissue as well. Upon being taken out of the coma, Jared found out his own body was betraying him. He was intubated for eight days, and was placed on a ventilator to help him breathe. He lost the ability to speak, and began losing control of his muscles. They would involuntarily twitch, and became hard to control. The top notch medical staff in Rochester treated him in the hospital for six weeks, where Jared lost 40 pounds. Jared had to retrain his body to gain back proper motor control, and is still undergoing intense speech therapy to recover his normal speech. In the six months following his release, Jared was put on high doses of steroids and underwent rigorous therapy, which he attacked with the same attitude he had when trying to prove his detractors wrong. He's also faced intense emotional stress, suffering from PTSD, and receiving treatment from a psychologist. When Jared ran into his old High School coach, he received a recommendation to join him at Light Speed CrossFit once he was cleared. A few weeks later, he decided to reach out to me.

Both he and his parents were a bit nervous, not knowing what to expect. Jared's father came and watched the foundations classes, and we'd speak after each class about his progress. Watching Jared move, you would never know what he had been through. His form was incredible right from the first class, and he processes coaching cues and makes corrections almost instantly. What also stands out is that his parents drive him to class every morning at 5:30AM. You could see the type of support he has received, and the reason for

130

the drive that is instilled in him. To go from being unsure if he would ever be able to function normally again, to finishing "Murph" and squatting 255lbs in just 7 months is amazing, and a testament to Jared's heart and desire. FYI – 255 is a lifetime squat PR.

In his own words, Jared said CrossFit has "basically changed my life, and I'm so thankful for the coach, Ryan, as he has helped push me past where I've ever been before physically and has also helped me to recover mentally in the form of an outlet. All of the anger, nervousness and intense anxiety is released when I'm at CrossFit; there I don't have time to think, which is just what I need. The experience has been great and the environment is awesome and very welcoming which is exactly what I've needed after being through what I've been through. CrossFit has helped me to regain sight of my goals and has brought me closer to them. There's a famous streetball basketball player by the name of Pat the Roc, who sent me a video recently saying to remember three letters, A.I.P. which stands for anything is possible. I have carried this message with me throughout this extremely difficult recovery and the challenges that have come along with it and it applies to all aspects of life." Watching Jared take off running makes me truly believe that anything is possible. *About the Author: Ryan Saraco, Head Coach at* Light Speed CrossFit*, has been a CrossFit trainer since 2012. He holds CrossFit Level 1 and Level 2 certificates. A former attorney, Ryan left the corporate world to pursue his true passion of helping people become the best possible versions of themselves through CrossFit.*

During one workout, the time cap was 20 minutes which meant that you did as much of the workout as you could in 20 minutes, but after the time was up you were supposed to stop. After everyone was done, I still had about 10 minutes left of work to finish my sets and I wasn't going to leave any stone unturned, so I finished it up, while the others watched in awe and cheered me on. The workouts pushed me and were always fun and rewarding.

Around this time I adopted a Paleo diet. This was in line with the theme of Crossfit, and others in the gym were doing it too. This meant no processed or "man made" foods, no dairy, and no grains. My goal in doing this, after much research, was to decrease inflammation naturally (although my intentions made sense, I have since learned that inflammation is a result of dis-ease and is actually part of the body's healing process, rather than the distinct cause of illness). I wanted to help my body "fight off" and heal from what remained of the illness, and was hoping to get it working smoothly. I was eating good quality meats, fruits and vegetables, along with healthy fats and a couple of paleo snacks, so overall a pretty solid diet. At the time, I believed that this would help to end the lasting effects of my "illness." But little did I understand how complicated it all was, or know how many more issues would arise, and how many more years it would take, and how much there was still left to learn about healing.

I loved the improvements I was making at Crossfit, as well as working out here also helped me deal with my anxiety. As I looked at it, if I had a heart attack, there were other people watching who would be aware and would take care of me. This was some of the irrational thinking my mind was doing at the time. When I was in the gym it was easy for me to block out everything else, so I could really focus on what I was doing. Also, the 2015 summer as I said earlier was so awesome and meant so much to me that I was worried about losing the people and never getting to see them again; so once again the gym was there to calm me down. But unfortunately the gym had to close since too many members had left, and the owner couldn't keep the gym open anymore.

For the rest of 2016, I followed an app for Crossfit workouts to do on my own. It wasn't the same, and also I didn't have a coach watching me or people to compete with. I still enjoyed it until I started getting hurt. I wasn't sure why this was happening to me considering how I took such good care of my body, but this was another mystery that would be solved later on. While still trying to take control over my health, I continued following the Paleo diet all through 2016 and through 2017.

INJURIES

MY MIND WANTED TO ADVANCE BUT MY BODY WASN'T READY

Chapter 27

Starting in high school, I began to get injured a lot, mostly with ankle sprains. And as I've learned with any problem, if you don't address the root cause, it will keep hurting you over and over again. So, in the summer after 11th grade as well as prior to/during my senior soccer and basketball seasons, I was spraining my ankles often (I could probably write a book about the causes of these injuries as I have since gained tons of training knowledge). Keep in mind my body was definitely under a lot of stress–I was in the midst of playing three sports, playing on multiple basketball and soccer teams, going on almost no sleep, and trying to weight train on top of all that. That's a ton of stress on the body. And to put it simply, my body couldn't handle the forces placed upon it, whether physically or emotionally. During my 11th grade summer, I was set to go to California for the Maccabi games with a new team who had asked me to play for them. I was playing really well on this team in these practices, and I was once again given the nickname "Nash." The day before leaving, we had a basketball practice and I was driving to the hoop when my foot locked under me leaving me with an awful sprain. My dad basically had to carry me to the car as we drove to the hospital. California was off—I was on crutches for a week and had physical therapy for the rest of the summer. (I would not think about missing camp though, of course!). Then, I kept reaggravating the injury over the next year because I would just put an ankle brace on it and wear more protective sneakers (which is not the right advice as I later learned). My ankles became extremely tight and immobile, which is not how they are meant to function. I also was unable to participate in the NYU basketball camp that I was invited to. I had another ankle injury to start my senior year of basketball and another one that impacted the start of my soccer season, and it hurt every time I ran.

Fast forward two years later...after much anticipation, the summer of 2015 finally came, and was super pivotal as you've read about. In the middle of that summer, we were playing soccer when my co-counselor throws the ball in, which was a bit too far behind me. Me, being the super competitor who acted like a camper, which is one of the things that all the kids loved about me, I tried to do a bicycle kick to score the goal. My foot got caught underneath me and I felt a crack. I was down. James immediately rushed over to me to make sure I was okay and was really worried for me. The other counselors helped me up and got me on a golf cart to the nurse's office. After some X-rays (which I have since learned carry dangers of their own due to radiation, especially when you get them often), it turned out to be another severe ankle sprain. This meant my awesome summer and favorite time of year, after my severe illness, was going to be altered. The next day I came into camp hobbling because I couldn't stand to not be there. James and my other boys were constantly checking on me, trying to help support and comfort me whenever I needed it. Thankfully, that was the only injury for that summer and while it hindered me a bit, I was able to make the most of my time at camp and continue to enjoy it to the fullest. Once again, I was being taught that life has no obligation to be fair, but that didn't mean I was gonna throw in the towel. I had to show others how I wouldn't let my "sickness" and now this injury destroy me. When the following summer rolled around, I continued trying to avoid the problems with my ankles while I braced them and acted as if there wasn't a deeper issue, which only resulted in more injuries. The next summer (2016) I believe I sprained each ankle 4 times, whether in my summer men's basketball league or at camp playing. Needless to say, that summer was not as enjoyable as I had hoped. During that summer I was sick (or as I like to say now—I was expressing symptoms...) with strep throat once and another "respiratory infection" (their words not mine), which the doctors yet again couldn't diagnose exactly. I just couldn't seem to avoid the "sickness" or the injury "bug." This was a foreboding of things to come. I didn't realize it at the time, but my body's systems and overall health were seriously compromised. I was nowhere near out of the woods as there were more underlying health issues lurking.

After that summer was over, the injuries started to pile up. Now, it wasn't just my ankles, but during my workouts I started to get back pain that got progressively worse. Soon, it got to the point where it felt like I was throwing my back out every time I lifted weights. My elbows and shoulders started hurting too. I couldn't even walk or sleep without feeling the pain. This became extremely frustrating and depressing. For a kid who always tried his hardest to be healthy and strong, and now couldn't even play sports or lift weights without pain, and couldn't even keep his body healthy, I felt defeated. I cried so many days and would argue with my parents in frustration. But, as you'll see me mention in other parts of the book, it seems that every time I'm at rock bottom and feel like I can't go on anymore, a healing guide or a sign appears in my life, and I'm reinvigorated with hope and motivation to keep going. I tried watching YouTube videos and people on Instagram and went to a bunch of doctors who were of zero use. The constant stretching only made things worse and put me in more pain. My favorite influencer on Instagram at the time was fitness/athlete Terron Beckham aka @fbaftermath, and I also followed his friend Matt Kido @gokuflex. Both of them were living in NYC. They each had posted videos with this guy who called himself the Bodmechanic. He supposedly could fix any injury and get you feeling better than ever. This was a glimmer of hope. So I tried to find him online to get an appointment. Unfortunately, first I found his old office. For some reason, the Bodmechanic's name (Andreas Saltas) and description were still on the website. We got to the office and I didn't see him there. We asked for Andreas and were told that he no longer works there. I discovered that he had opened up his own practice. I figured the office must use the same techniques and probably has the same knowledge that he does. So, I did a bunch of sessions there with the classic trained therapist, the ones who have 10 patients at a time. He did some muscle stim, gave me some ice and a couple of exercises. After my sessions that were covered by insurance were up and I wasn't feeling any better, the therapist suggested that I go for an MRI. The doctors told me that I had something called "congenital lumbar stenosis."

Learning of this felt like a needle going through my body and my athletic dreams. When I told this therapist "my diagnosis" he said to me,

"Well, you can't lift weights or do any strenuous activity anymore." So I immediately started tearing up and said, "Well how am I ever going to dunk or play basketball if I can't lift weights?" His response to me was, "Now all of a sudden you're an athlete? You want to be a basketball player and a powerlifter?" I left his office totally discouraged and depressed. This guy obviously didn't know anything about me or how to help me. He didn't know my story and that I don't take no for an answer. When I came home and laid down on the couch crying, my dad started telling me that maybe I didn't have to lift weights and that I would be fine. When he realized that I wasn't going to accept this, he finally said to me, "If you want to be able to lift weights and dunk a basketball, I know you'll find a way." That came in the form of continuing my quest for this guy who they called Bodmechanic. When I showed his page to my parents on Instagram, they thought this guy was a witch doctor and that he would hurt me. As I talked about early on, my parents are often (in my view) way overprotective. In their defense, throughout my life while looking for ways to improve myself, I had sometimes been a very gullible kid who would fall for marketing schemes easily. As my nana likes to say I'm not gullible, I'm just overly trusting. But I was persistent with this. Although I can be overly trusting, I also can read people really well and know a good thing when I see it, and I knew that if anyone could help me heal my body, this was the guy. I finally convinced my parents to contact his office at his new location, Human Fitness, and was given a warning from my parents that if this doesn't work, it's on me. One thing I've discovered is that when you don't do things the conventional way, you also have to accept the risk of the blame coming down on you when things go wrong. I guess that's how society works because when you just go along with conventional thinking, you absolve yourself of responsibility and have a built in excuse: "I was just following the 'experts'" or "I was just doing what I was told." So we got an appointment at the end of December 2016. When I first met Andreas, I was blown away and incredibly intrigued. I actually couldn't keep the smile off my face while he was educating me on what it would take for me to heal. I told him my whole story about my life threatening illness and a bond began, which I wouldn't completely understand why, until later on. Whenever I learn something that really piques my interest and will benefit me, I get this big goofy smile on my face and sometimes even start to laugh (in addition to the fact that due to my neurological problems, I was also laughing at the wrong times occasionally anyway). The reason I mention our unspoken bond is because I learned that he was in a motorcycle accident when he was about my age and he was paralyzed for some time, and by miracles and hard work he survived and learned to walk again. He remembered everything that his physical therapists had done for him and wanted to give back and become the best therapist in the world. So, he was taken aback when he heard my story and we related to each other.

Back to the treatment: When I showed him the MRI he basically tossed it out the window and told me with the utmost confidence that the MRI was the doctors' cop out so that everyone could give up on me. But he wouldn't. He asked me if I had any textbooks. I replied, "I have a lot since I'm in college." His first piece of advice was to put 1 or 2 of them under my feet while sitting down as a way of helping me engage the right muscles while seated— and I cracked up when he said, "You're not gonna need those textbooks anyway." (LOL) He demonstrated to me that he was going to do everything he could to help me restore my body, but it was going to require a lot of work on my end too. It wasn't some magic pill that he was going to give me; it required me to put the work in! He knew that I was an athlete and wanted to get back to lifting weights and even when I told him my large goals, he was encouraging and would help me achieve them. He blew me away with his knowledge, and to this day I view him as probably the smartest person I know when it comes to the human body from a physical standpoint. Andreas' knowledge is unparalleled, and to go along with his caring and amazingly kind demeanor, he is a member of my team who I am so grateful to have!

It was not an easy road to get my body back to 100%. When they say that knowledge is power, they leave out the part about how important it is to be able to apply that knowledge. Andreas and I had to work tirelessly. We started with an appointment once every 1-2 weeks because most of the healing was achieved by me doing my homework. I was a model patient as he would tell me and his other patients. I trusted him and did everything to the best of my ability. He gave me breathing exercises and exercises to strengthen muscles I never even knew I had. He worked on my lifting form and gave me numerous cues to focus on. Later on, he would implement visual training as well as balance training and joint end range of motion mobility exercises to do constantly every day (which I still do). He even gave me tools to reduce the damage that my "illness complications" caused to my body (such as the way the "illness" created improper breathing patterns and excessive stress on certain organs). His learning is never done as his experience continues to grow. That inspires me to never stop learning. It took about a year before I truly felt pain free, but I got there once all the education he gave me finally set in. This was true learning taking place and was going to be lifelong knowledge that would help me through my athletic career, and even more, I could use it to help others. I was always curious and constantly asking more questions. Towards the end of the summer of 2017, I was squatting pain free and deadlifting too, along with all of my other lifts, as well as playing basketball and soccer and running pain free again. My strength numbers were going up and I was finally able to jump again, so I could resume my dunk journey. Nothing worth having comes easy and there is no quick fix that is permanent, but you have to stick with it. As I've said before, it's okay to cry and okay to be frustrated and depressed, but it's never okay to give up. As I like to say, if you stay in the game long enough, you will either get what you want or something even better.

Speaking of using this knowledge to help others, I have been able to help James heal his elbow and ankle injuries by applying what I had learned. He has adopted the same mobility routine. And he has since used that knowledge to help some of his school friends, so we created a positive chain reaction. James thought I was doing some magic, just as I thought when I first met Andreas. I then went on to help my mom with her elbow issues too, and have even put out some YouTube videos of my own with this knowledge. I would always do the exercises with the people I was helping to show full support. That's what life is about though, finding solutions to your own problems and then helping others through your experience. This was my way of paying it forward. Plus I have continued my learning about the body every day with my own experimentation and by watching and interacting with many helpful podcasts and videos.

DON'T GIVE UP DON'T EVER GIVE UP

Chapter 28

"I know all about giving up, and what scares me is that it's easy." (Vinny Paz in *Bleed for This*). That's the truth. Most people give up because that is the easy way out. It takes no effort to quit and throw in the towel. It is scary and it's tempting to give up because of the fact that it's so easy. Success isn't easy, in anything. Nothing worth having comes easy. You gotta be willing to fight for it. I had to fight for my life, fought for every breath at one point, and built myself up from the depths of life. There were a ton of times when giving up seemed like the logical solution to get out of my problems, but I couldn't do it. Quitting was not an option. I had to show myself that I am stronger than anything life throws at me, I was going to trust God's massive plans for me, and show others that I wasn't giving up—I was gonna put my all into this fight.

NYU Basketball Tryout-The Final Opportunity to Play College Basketball

And my story was far from over yet. I had to start from scratch, as I was recovering from the depths of my challenging health circumstances and used all the fight in me to get me back onto the court. Once I really got back into playing basketball, my goal was to become better than ever before, revamp my training, and literally transform into the best version of myself. In 2016, I started playing in a men's basketball league (as I was doing with soccer at the time too). The competition consisted of many former college and high school players. A few games in, I had a game to remember. First half, I drop 22 points and finished with 28 in only about 20 minutes of playing time. The same kid who was in a coma a year and a half earlier, who was told he might not make it, who couldn't reach the rim a year prior, was back to getting buckets. After I had been at NYU for a year (which you'll read about in the next chapter), I was trying to get onto the NYU team, so we hired a guy to film a couple of my games as game tape to send to the coach. In one of these games I had a triple double with 24 points, 12 rebounds, and 10 assists, and I hit the game winning last second shot. This was the comeback in motion, still years away from feeling all better and from having recovered from my health

140

issues, but this was showing how I fight. I sent my tape to the NYU coach who invited me to first join the team in some private scrimmages and then a tryout a few weeks later. In these team scrimmages, I guess the kids really don't like the idea of a walk-on taking their spot, so I would barely touch the ball, which was really disheartening. Most of the players wouldn't even look my way no matter how open I was. Then, in between games we had to shoot to see who got to play in the next game. If any of you have ever tried taking a 3 pointer as your first shot of the day, you know how hard it is. So after playing a full game where I was basically just running up and down the court, not having taken a shot all day, I step up and airball a 3 pointer (also keep in mind that my elbow injury had been creeping up so it would often hurt when I would shoot). I walked back from the gym that day crying. I felt humiliated in front of all these players. I knew I was good enough to play on this team, but nobody was giving me a chance or any encouragement. I spoke with my parents on the phone who told me not to give up. Whatever happens happens, but in the end, at least I'll say I tried my best and gave it my all. I wiped away the tears and came back again a few days later. This time I had a bit of time to warm up and play in a game with some of the students not on the team, and I was making every shot, crossing guys up, putting the ball between their legs, and making sweet passes. I tried to bring myself back to having FUN with the game I love by taking the pressure off. Then, I get into the game with the NYU players. First play of the game, a kid on my team basically gave the ball to the other team on a pass, but I ripped the ball from the player and put it up and scored. Then a few plays later, the player I was guarding drives by me thinking he has an open lane. I caught up to him and pinned (blocked) his shot off the backboard and drove the ball up the court and got an assist. I had another block a few plays later, and although I still basically got zero passes thrown my way, I was laying it all on the line. Then, when we were shooting for teams, this time I made the three pointer. I felt a bit better this time walking back to class. It may not have been an ideal situation and it was certainly socially uncomfortable, being the kid who knows no one on the team and has a speech "disorder" and is also (as per usual) the smallest player on the court, but I wasn't stopping.

Then came the tryout. I was really nervous. I felt like this was my last chance to achieve the dream of playing college basketball like I had set out to do as a little kid. My dad drove me into the city and told me that no matter what, he knows I'm worthy of playing college ball and just to show them everything I got, take my shots (as he's been telling me for years now), and whatever happens, happens. Coach Warren called me earlier to give me some encouragement as well and to tell me how proud he is of me for doing this. I get to the tryout with all the same kids there who wouldn't look my way during the past few weeks. I did some breathing techniques to calm down, as well as some visualization. Myself and the other walk-on hopefuls would be trying out in a team practice. I played some of the best basketball I ever had. Throughout the whole tryout I shot somewhere between 75-90% on 3 pointers, layups, reverse layups, made the correct reads, and played hard defense. One play, the coach set up a trap where I was supposed to go around a screen and get trapped by two guys. I reject the screen, crossover and take it all the way to the hoop for a layup, making the kids look silly as they chased me down trying to block my shot. Then another play we're doing a 1 v 1 drill where you had a 3 dribble limit. I was going up against a kid who was 7'1 tall! First time around I tried to drive by him but he caught up to me and blocked my shot. Next time I swish a 3 right in his face. Then, during the shooting drills we started from mid range catch and shoot, then moved onto 3 pointers catch and shoot, as well as off the dribble. Out of about 15 shots, I missed only 2 or 3 total. Then we did some fast break drills 3 on 2 then 2 on 1; I sank 4 out of 5 shots during this. By the end of the tryout the kids on the team were high fiving me and complimenting me by name. I had earned their respect. It came time to go into the coaches room and hear whether or not I made it. I was sure I made it. How could I not have? In my head, I was preparing for the team schedule but I had also decided that no matter what, I proved to myself that I was at the level where I could play college basketball and at the very least I had made an incredible comeback thus far. Then, an interesting thought popped into my head. For once, I was going to truly surrender the outcome. I controlled everything that I could and all the hours upon hours of work I put in, and had an unbelievable tryout and proved everyone wrong again who said I was never going to be good enough to play college basketball.

And more importantly, to work my way back to this point was an accomplishment in and of itself. So at this point, if I don't make it, I'm at peace with that.

I walked into the coach's office with his assistants there too. The coach first tells me he knows my dad's cousin Spanky who coaches high school basketball and was a tremendous player himself. I thought this was a good sign, but then he tells me I didn't make the team. He didn't take any walk-ons as he said his team was set. Me trying to be the respectful and kind person I am, I shook all their hands and thanked them for letting me tryout. As much as it killed me to do it, I was in a good mood because of how well I did in the tryout. I said to the coach, "What can I do to get better?" And the coach hesitates for a minute and says "Just uh everything." It was in that moment that I knew he either hadn't watched the tryout or just didn't care enough to help me out, as he had his mind set beforehand that he wouldn't take me. *Incidentally, a year or two later he got fired.*

Truthfully, I wasn't mad or bitter though. I had done what I came to do, proved to myself and everyone else who doubted me that my hard work meant something, and that I had done everything I could to make me the best player I could be. I walked out to the car with a big smile on my face as I told my dad everything that happened, and he was extremely proud of me. The crazy part is it didn't matter that I didn't make the team, it didn't matter that I was never going to play college basketball. Everything I had done to get to this point was all a part of my transformation and leveling up as a person. And the offers in high school, the excellent performances at these college tryouts, and where my game is today, that was enough to show me what I'm capable of. And even had none of that happened, even if I didn't receive any external approval, I knew that I learned more about my own inner self—that I had that grit and stuff that couldn't be taught—and you couldn't take that away from me. I proved to myself and to all the other underdogs as well as the haters that anything is possible, and you couldn't tell me otherwise. The journey doesn't always go as planned, but if you're open to it, you wind up learning a whole lot more along the way about who you are and what you

can accomplish with hard work and dedication and a promise to yourself
to never give up. That same kid who was in a coma and on a ventilator
and feeding tube and fighting for his life in 4 different hospitals over 6
weeks and would need another 9+ years to recover; the same kid who was
told he was too small to ever accomplish anything athletically, whose
anxiety crippled him before games over the years—he was a better player
than ever before. And even though I was still far away from being done
with my severe health problems and from overtaking the biggest challenge
of my life in completing my healing process, I knew I still had a lot more
living to do, and I would eventually be my best self in all areas of my life.

Back to Soccer 2015-2017

At the day camp we always played a lot of soccer, and as a counselor,
especially when you're like me who does things with the passion and
fervor of a camper, some of us really go all out and the kids loved that.
During the summer of 2015, our group was often playing games with one
of the groups whose group leader was a soccer specialist the previous
year. And after watching me play a bunch, he was impressed and also
inspired by my story. He asked me if I wanted to join his men's league
soccer team which was very competitive and was full of former college
players and even 2 former semi pro players. I loved the idea as this was a
great way for me to prove to myself how good I could be as a soccer
player, and just to compete at a high level to show myself how much
better I had actually gotten since my illness (even though I was still far
from healed yet). Just as with everything in my life, I had to prove myself
to the team. I wasn't gonna be given a handout just because of everything
I had been through. The first few games were a difficult adjustment. I was
the youngest one on the team. During this time, I would hear some talk
from my teammates wondering if I could handle this level of play. Then, I
slowly gained respect from the other players who would commend my
work ethic on the field. I started to adjust to the tough gameplay and kept
improving. Although I started off with limited minutes of playing time, I
eventually became a big contributor. Then, one day we found out that our
goalie was quitting, so once again I offered to step up. This generated
even more respect from my teammates as they were always telling the
team that we need more players like Jared. The main captain started

calling me after games to tell me how well I played. In the team email, there were times throughout the seasons when the other captains would tell everyone how admirable my effort was and how committed I was to the team. I helped our team to a bunch of wins and performed at a super high level. I was better than I had ever been before in a lot of ways. Regardless of my performance, even being back on the field was an accomplishment. And of course my dad was there for every game, even in the games when it was hailing, snowing, and pouring rain. That's what it means to persevere—to go through everything I have and to come back better than ever before. The work wasn't done yet, but I showed myself what I was capable of, as well as everyone who doubted what I could do as an athlete. Unfortunately, towards the end of our 2017 season, players started quitting and the team ultimately broke up. Even though I'm not currently on a team, I still love to play and work on my skills to go along with my other athletic pursuits and may try to find another team in the future. I recently set a new PR on how many juggles in a row with over 220, and my skills are more refined than ever.

COLLEGE- HOFSTRA AND NYU (2015)

Chapter 29

After my brief stint at Cornell and losing that semester, I still had planned on going back the next semester. At the last possible second, the night before we were supposed to head back up to school, I called an audible. I decided there was no way I was ready to be away from my family after the hell I had just gone through. I was not in the right state of mind emotionally and my speech was barely understandable, so this scared me thinking about what I would encounter if I were hundreds of miles from home. I wasn't even off the steroids medication yet, so I made the tough, yet wise decision to go to school locally for a semester. I was well enough to do a semester at Hofstra University, about 20 minutes from my house. As much as I was opposed to school in general and the whole system as I'll talk more about, I actually didn't mind this semester. I only took two classes, but one of my professors was really great and we got along well, and the other class wasn't too bad either. It was definitely kind of a low key experience, but that was what I needed at the time. I wasn't ready to go back full speed and was still recovering both physically and emotionally, and everything I did was so draining. Then after my awesome and much needed summer of 2015, once again I had a decision to make. I couldn't extend my health leave of absence from Cornell much longer. If it were totally up to me, I actually would've preferred to stay at Hofstra (or drop out completely if I'm being totally honest lol). But my parents wanted me to either go back to Cornell or transfer to NYU, as NYU had a health and dietetics program which was more similar to Cornell's. I still didn't feel ready to be away from home and still had a lot more recovery work to do, so I reluctantly agreed to go to NYU. I spent the next 4 years there. And to be honest, without trying to be too negative, I really hated most of it. By the end of my time there, I was so fed up with the whole school system and teachers who I felt weren't teaching the right way. I always thought that college was supposed to be a place where you were encouraged to do your own research on topics that you felt were pertinent to your growth as a person and to your career. I never felt comfortable in offering any of my own opinions that did not agree with those that were taught. Maybe that's just the way college is

146

these days in general. Aside from a few friendly kids and my very kind advisers, I really just felt that this was not a good fit for me. It was a lonely experience. Although occasionally I would speak with a few nice classmates during school where we would share some laughs, there were no friends with whom I would hang out, outside of class. I couldn't wait to get out and go home as soon as I arrived. One of the positive moments at NYU was the amazing basketball tryout in 2016. The only real enjoyable times I had were when my mom would come in to have lunch with me at Hu Kitchen or Springbone (2 delicious Paleo/ancestral based restaurants). Other than that, in between classes I typically sat in the park or in a building on campus and just kept to myself, listening to music or reading a book or texting my parents or friends from home. To make matters worse, I was also going through severe digestive issues and speech issues during my last two years. And since I didn't want to live there, I had to take the train in every day which was an exhausting hour and a half commute both ways. Once I finished up, I told myself that was the last time I would let others decide what I'm doing with my life. I wanted to make my parents happy as always, so I wasn't going to quit and didn't really have much of a choice either. So I bit the bullet and graduated in 2019 with a degree in Nutrition and Dietetics. This was an amazing accomplishment and I'm not knocking it at all. To go through what I went through and to still finish up college only a semester late was pretty amazing. It's just that I was even more bitter about the whole school experience, and I personally don't really feel that a degree is a strong measure of actual knowledge and intelligence (however, of course there are certain professions where having a degree is essential based on the way society is set up). There were also many additional factors involved. First off, my original college plan and original athletics goals all fell apart. This was not where I was "supposed to be." On top of all that, I felt like my opinions just weren't being heard or valued in classes. Many days I would leave feeling enraged due to the professors quieting me and shutting me out when I expressed an opinion or belief different from the curriculum. And of course, my health was not in a good state, which made things even more uncomfortable. For some, college is supposed to be the "best 4 years of your life." I never really bought into that because if that's the best time, then what is there to look forward to for the rest of your life? There are so many more real, and in my opinion, better pleasures out there beyond what most college kids think of. But of course some people do love it and to each their own. Maybe it just wasn't for me. I'm not the "party" kid type as I prefer the company of a small number of people whom I choose. Furthermore, I prefer to research the subjects that I want to learn about on my own. I prefer to seek the truth on topics rather than be taught what to believe. I'm that guy trying to break free from the "matrix" and have done even way more questioning in recent years. So maybe that's just how it was for someone like me.

Thankfully I was living at home, so I compartmentalized school from my home life. Therefore, after some really grueling days, I was still able to have fun and amazing times once I came home.

MY THOUGHTS ON SCHOOL...BEING SELF-MOTIVATED WILL GET YOU FURTHER THAN ANYTHING YOU WILL LEARN IN THE CLASSROOM

Chapter 30

To start my thoughts on school I should first put in this quote, "How you do one thing is the way you do everything." People often assume that I must have loved school considering my achievements and how many hours I put into studying. This couldn't be farther from the truth. I love working hard to complete tasks and proving people wrong who doubt what I'm capable of, as I am ultra competitive. Don't get me wrong—I absolutely love learning, but I love learning the truth and exploring topics on a much deeper level rather than the topics that get chosen for me and that are full of falsehoods as I've since learned from doing my own research. I don't like being told what to think and how to feel. However, I still gave school my absolute all and wanted to be the smartest in every class and would spend hours upon hours every night studying. I couldn't do something and not give it my all. However, I strongly believe that self-motivated learning promotes the best learning experience for you, better than school ever could, because it allows you to become your own teacher. Only you know the best way for you to learn. And to be honest, once you're done with school, it takes a lot of "unlearning" to arrive at real truths. School should not be the end of your learning because there are so many resources available these days and we should all be taking advantage of them. For instance, when it came to starting up my YouTube channel and growing all of my social media, as I've mentioned in the past, I had no prior experience with filmmaking. I had no idea how to use a camera or video editing software, but I had a desire to spread my message to the world on a bigger platform. So, I essentially taught myself how to do it all with the help of testing things out as well as watching online tutorials, and within a few months I think I was making some pretty awesome videos and am constantly leveling up. It takes a lot of work, dedication, and discipline, but if you want something bad enough you'll find a way.

Moreover, all of the stress put on me and stress that I put on myself to achieve in school impacted my life as a whole and contributed to my anxiety. This took away from other healthy aspects of my life. Sacrifices had to be made, and discipline was never a problem for me. It wasn't all for naught considering that I had numerous academic achievements of which I'm extremely proud, but what does it all mean? We are always told that we will need to learn this piece of information for the next level, but does any of it ever matter in our lives? Do test scores really matter in the long run? (Just to clarify I'm not talking about education in general…I'm talking about the Rockefeller education system and the way it's designed.) Unfortunately, I believe that a lot of our education system is set up to deter outside the box thinkers and keep the diverse minds tamed. It's set up to indoctrinate kids into believing the "accepted way of thinking" and to teach everyone to be the same. It's set up to make you okay with constantly being busy with trivial tasks, so this way you never stop to question what our real purpose on this earth is. When a kid comes in with a different way of thinking and can't sit still, they get labeled with learning disabilities that follow them their whole lives and sometimes even get medicated. A lot of times, they just learn differently and have more energy that could be used positively in other areas. We can talk about all of the nefarious reasons as to why the system is set up as it is, I believe, such as trying to keep people more docile and more easily controlled. But for now I want to offer some solutions. Also, generally speaking as I'm sure many of us can attest to, sitting down for 8 hours a day when you are a kid with endless energy is very boring and isn't how humans are meant to function, when meanwhile research has shown that having fun helps you retain more information. Of course some teachers do a good job of making learning fun, but I believe there should be more emphasis on this. Learning should be fun, or at the very least more exciting and more interactive. Moreover, a school setting isn't right for everyone—I believe especially these days, homeschooling should be encouraged much more often when feasible, based on the level of indoctrination that currently goes into public schooling. Of course socialization is very important, as

150

well as getting involved in activities such as sports, music, and clubs, so these skills should be prioritized no matter what education setting you're in. Also, there is something to be said for learning to respect your elders and respect others, but I believe this should come more from the parents. However, many government policies center around getting parents to give up their kids to the government funded schools, and the kids will learn whatever the government wants them to. I believe that's all backwards—the parent or parents should have more of a say in what the child learns. But in the cases where this can't be done, schools should be teaching more critical thinking and thinking for the students. The goal should not be obedience to the information; there should be room for diversity of thought and opinion. There also needs to be more emphasis on learning through experience. As I mentioned, I am someone who was never satisfied with hearing "well that's the answer because that's just the way it is." I always had to go deeper and ask more questions until I got to the bottom of it (Which I guess explains why I began finding more truth in the "conspiracy truther world" as I call it, rather than that of the "experts." When enough things don't add up and you're told not to question them, that never sat right with me.) This is where experience and your own perceptions come into play. You can't fully learn something unless you feel and experience it to the fullest. All this teaching for the test doesn't actually make people smarter; it makes them better test takers and better subjects. For instance, I have had a lot of success in recent years learning through podcasts and YouTube videos. When I listen to these people keeping things interesting and relating it to real life rather than just listening for what I'll need to know on a test, this helps me retain more information. For some professions, the school you get into definitely helps you to go farther in that field, as that's the way the game of life is currently set up. But, if you're someone who is trying to carve out your own niche, school is a means to an end. They will also try to tell you that college is where it all matters. "That is where you will learn the bulk of what you want to do." But, I found it to be the same as all of the prior education, if not worse, when it came to being taught things that I would later discover to not be true. I always knew that I didn't want to use college to build my career and lifestyle. I would be self-motivated to learn and to work on myself and my skills to get me where I wanted to go.

While I always had these feelings, they deeply intensified after getting sick and realizing how little these test scores actually matter in your life.

School has you stay seated for 8 hours a day while listening to their points of views on subjects that they consider important, and on top of that hours of homework (which was originally only supposed to be used as punishment). If you have a different point of view, they basically tell you tough luck, listen to us anyway. School teaches you how to be like everybody else. So many teachers and professors, whether they will admit to it or not, have a bias with the information they are teaching. (Yes, schools have agendas that they're supposed to conform to and are paid by the government to do so.) It's so important to be able to think for yourself and learn on your own. The best teachers are the ones who give you the TOOLS to think for yourself so that you come up with your own conclusions. You search up the data, find the facts and form opinions based on what you find, rather than have someone tell you what you are supposed to believe or how you're supposed to think.

QUESTIONING EVERYTHING TO REACH THE HARD UNPOPULAR TRUTHS

Before diving into my next topic, I want to share about a story my mom used to read to me growing up called *How Joe The Bear and Sam The Mouse Got Together*. This story was about two totally different people/animals...they ate different foods, liked different things, and had totally different lives. But at the end of every day, they could still meet up and have ice cream. Now, I'm not saying we have to be best friends with every person who has different beliefs from us, but can we at least be respectful towards others?

I am someone who tries my best to spread peace, love, and positivity among everyone. However, from a young age, I have always questioned everything I have been taught. I have never accepted lessons taught to me simply because I was told—I would look at every angle of the simplest lesson and dissect it until I reasoned in my own way and formed my own conclusions. I believe that every individual is entitled to their own opinion on any matter—and these differing opinions should be heard and considered and discussed. Isn't that the best way to learn? It is so important to remember that everyone is coming from a different place and has their own thoughts and interpretations. So just because someone may not see things the same way I do, this doesn't mean I should think less of them as long as they are a good kind person. As human beings, I feel it is incumbent upon us to have respect for *everyone*, as well as not impose our beliefs on others or shut others down because they feel differently from you. (Of course many of you who either follow me on social media or have watched my Rabbit Hole Roundups or Hard Truths videos/podcasts already know much of what I am about to say. But this is more for the people who don't already know this about me.) The purpose of me sharing is not to stir controversy for the sake of stirring controversy, but rather to open your minds to topics you may have never been exposed to. Also, as you will see and I will go into depth on, these beliefs have empowered me greatly and helped me understand how truly amazing we are so I hope you can come in with an open mind and use these to empower yourselves as well! What I believe has been hidden from us the most is our own divinity…

Why don't we learn about those who sought to give us free energy and demonstrated that we actually live in a world of abundance, not scarcity of resources? Until we learn the truth about history, things like MK Ultra and Operation Paperclip amongst many other government operations, HAARP, chemtrails (watch Matt Landman's movie *Frankenskies* for an in depth analysis), our existence, the incredible healing powers within our own bodies amongst many other things that I have questioned—the education system will always feel flawed. Why can't we question the dangers of vaccines which I believe are totally unnecessary and actually harmful for anyone who researches the ingredients in them, as well as the lack of proof for the existence of viruses? Why is it considered "essential" for everyone to inject heavy metals and many other harmful chemical ingredients (formaldehyde, PEG, aborted fetal cells, etc.) into our bodies in the name of "health?" Could the reason why they push germ theory be that it means different medicines for every "germ"/"disease?" And as I've come to understand, symptoms from the body are how the body heals and detoxifies; so by stopping the symptoms are we just pushing the toxicity deeper into the body and trading acute illness for chronic disease?

Why can't we discuss what really happens with every false flag event? Why weren't we taught that NASA was founded by Werner Von Braun who came to the U.S. as part of Operation Paperclip? And working alongside him was Jack Parsons, L. Ron Hubbard, and Walt Disney (I suggest looking into each of their personal pasts). Do we even know what the moon actually is? How can the Sun and Moon both be out at the same time if as we are taught, "The moonlight is just a reflection of the Sun?" Could it actually be that the moon was placed within the firmament to be a light for the nighttime? And even if it were possible to land on the moon (which I don't believe it is), had they actually done it in 1969, why haven't we been back there since? Are we allowed to ask why we send billions of tax dollars every year to NASA and where this money actually goes? (For a really interesting explanation on the topic, I would recommend listening to the song *Stanley Kubrick* by B.o.B as well as his whole Elements album...also Eddie Bravo and Sam Tripoli and myself often cover these concepts on our podcasts) Can we ask why all images of the Earth are CGI-computer generated images? And why was there never any mention of dinosaurs prior to the mid 1800s? Could dinosaurs have actually been dragons or other megafauna that lived alongside humans rather than living billions of years ago as they want us to believe? I also believe that many of these big bones they find are actually evidence of Giants who were here in recent times. And speaking of which, who built all these massive structures in the 1700s and 1800s that they tell us were built with the extent of the technology being horse and buggy? Could these have been built by Nephilim or their descendants? Were there past resets that might have wiped out our true history and technology? Did they teach any of you in school that Rockefeller paid off the scientists at the Geneva convention to classify oil as a "fossil fuel" as a way of making it sound scarce and therefore could be profited heavily off of, when in fact oil (as well as water) regenerates in the Earth? As B.o.B says in his song *Bobiverse*, "Bones don't turn to oil." What proof is there that we are on a "spinning ball" which they claim spins at 1000 mph and moves through space they say at 66,000 miles per hour yet we don't feel any of this? If all that were true, we wouldn't see the same stars every night. How come the North Star-Polaris never moves? Could it be that maybe we're actually on a flat plane surrounded by massive ice walls (or even possibly a hollow Earth), and the firmament is dividing us from the heavens as the Bible says? That's what I believe. (Some great resources when it came to learning about flat Earth/true Earth/Biblical Earth have been Sean Hibbeler's films *Level, The Next Level* and *Level With Me.* You can also check out my awesome podcast episodes with Sean Hibbeler, as well as those with my new friend Tyler Hansen aka Fittest Flat Earther, Josh Monday, and others I've done and will do on the subject. Other great resources include Eddie Bravo's "Look Into It" podcast, "The Flat Earth Files" podcast, and the work of David Weiss-no relation to me lol). And as I spoke about with Chance Garton when he came on my podcast, first establishing what something is not, is actually super powerful in arriving at truth. Similarly, as Dr. Tom Cowan says it's about stripping down everything that is not true, and you will be left with what is. Furthering this point, what happened during Operation Fishbowl and Operation Dominic? Water always finds its level. It does not bend! A sextant, which is a tool that's been used by sailors to calculate distance between objects for many years, requires a triangle with 2 flat sides to work…this would not work on a spinning ball! Also, we can see too far…objects that are supposedly dipping below the curve aren't actually; they are just moving beyond our vision as evidenced by using simple technology and cameras to zoom in. Did you know that gravity has never actually been proven? Why do they claim it's strong enough to hold in all of Earth's waters, but it can't hold down a balloon or birds or even us down? (Look into electrostatics, density and buoyancy.) And why did basically every country who supposedly hates each other all agree to sign the Antarctic treaty? Why are we largely prohibited from traveling to Antarctica beyond the 60th parallel (outside of a tiny peninsula where there are penguins, or one of 2 islands-Rothschild Island or Deception Island)? Why don't we learn about how Admiral Byrd encountered other beings beyond the ice wall or how Captain Cook charted 60,000 miles of land in Antarctica? You might be saying to yourself, why would they lie to us about the shape of the Earth or who cares whether it's flat or round? But I believe the reason for the globe lie/deception and big bang hoax along with just about every other lie we've been taught, is all about promoting a worldview that disconnects us from God. And it's not so much the shape of the Earth that makes us divine and special creatures or not, but when you look into these things and realize that we didn't just randomly arrive here and didn't land here by accident and that we are living on God's creation, it empowers me and makes me realize my divine purpose here and that I chose to be here and that God granted me free will to manifest amazing things! Going along these same lines, could this idea of "evolution" be to convince us that we are here by accident and that we aren't as special and divine as I believe we are? They have never been able to show any legit evidence of species jumps. And if we really evolved from monkeys/apes, why are there no monkey fossils? Why don't we see a pig turning into a bird lol? Have you ever stopped to think about how crazy this concept actually sounds or did you just accept it because the teacher said so? How do they call it freedom when we pay in some cases half of our hard earned money to the government (which ends up being laundered or going to other countries for ridiculous causes or to line their own pockets) just to stay out of prison? I believe that every war is fought for the big bankers—they always profit off of war. Could another reason for these wars be to erase history and destroy historical artifacts such as star gates and remnants of old empires that we never learn about? What about the illusion of competition? Did you know that just about every big company is owned by either Blackrock, Vanguard, or State Street? They don't want us believing our own eyes…they just want us believing whatever they tell us. That's why they're always creating these "invisible enemies," to make you think that only they can see and handle them. Are we actually "free" if we can't ask these questions and share these beliefs without being censored? Have you ever looked into Tavistock Institute and the truth about the CIA and how they do social engineering aka brainwashing of the masses? Why can't we talk about the darkness and satanic agendas/freemasonry/occultism/Moloch worship in Hollywood and the music industry and even pro sports!? (This doesn't mean we can't ever enjoy their products and that we can't watch movies and pro sports games, because of course they are fun and enjoyable and we do need a break from the craziness of the world. And as I often say, just because the "ruling class" has one agenda, doesn't mean we can't flip the script and use these things for positive purposes. But it's important to be aware of the agendas and energy sucking purposes behind the "breads and circuses." Former pro football player Larry Johnson often speaks about a lot of these concepts on his social media.) Larry Johnson even takes it as far as to say that all pro sports are scripted and he does show some compelling evidence using gematria. I'm not sure whether I believe ALL of the players themselves are "in on it" and I don't agree with everything he says, but I also never count anything out. My personal thought is at the very least, can we see how they might be manipulated (especially the biggest games) to get certain results? These industries are multi billion dollar ENTERTAINMENT industries, and legally as I've learned from the book *The Fix Is Still In* by Brian Tuohy, they have no obligation to provide fans with honest outcomes. Do you think there is no desire for certain results to happen? Once again, this doesn't mean you can't still enjoy watching games or movies or listening to music…as one of my favorite IG accounts to follow @electric_being often says, "Be in the world, not of the world," which comes from the Bible. And I believe we can separate the art from the artist. Take all of this however you will, and if you think I'm crazy for asking these questions…so be it. I would also highly suggest watching many of my videos or podcasts on these subjects. Or if you are one of my younger readers who I hope to be inspiring and none of this makes sense to you, that's okay too lol. I hope the rest of the book can give you the inspiration you are looking for. I'm just trying to get people to realize how many beliefs are actually ours and have been proven to be true, versus how many are we just told to accept as truth because an authority figure told us it was! I'm not claiming to have all the answers, and I also feel it's important to not be overly consumed with and focus too much of our energy on the darkness because then we become the darkness. However, by knowing all this, we can then bring light to the situations, or even humor, as RJ and I like to do on our Rabbit Hole Roundup episodes lol. But until we are allowed to question everything without being shot down, gaslighted, censored/shadowbanned on social media or called crazy, and labeled a "conspiracy theorist," we will never have a solid foundation for our education system. I fully believe that one of the main reasons why I went through everything that I did is because in addition to being the perfect person to show people what's possible, I am also able to wake people up and get them asking these questions as well! Moreover, I believe that whatever beliefs (when it comes to the things that we have no legitimate direct proof of) empower you most and make you your best self who's kind and compassionate to others, those are what you should roll with. As I'll get into later, many of these beliefs have connected me more with spirituality and God, and so I feel super empowered when I dive into these rabbit holes. And that's the point I'm trying to make here with all these questions; I don't want anyone to live in more fear or in constant fear of this "boogeyman" who's out to get you. But rather, when you understand all of the lies and deception, you actually might, at least I have, come to understand how unstoppable we are and how much power we possess! And we all possess this divine spark even though "they" want to try so hard to disconnect us from God and from our true nature! So that is why I love questioning all prior beliefs and looking into all of these "conspiracy truths" as I'll call them, and I hope you have been able to gain this same understanding. And as a result, I believe once we understand this, we see that even the "controllers" or "ruling class" have a purpose that can be used for good. In this world of duality, by finally understanding all that we've been lied about, we can now explore the truth both about ourselves and this incredibly interesting world. By seeing all of the constraints that have been placed on us so that we don't see how amazing we are, we can break free and finally actualize our limitless potential, and that's what I want you guys to be able to take away from this or any of my videos on such topics!

(And to be clear, I have nothing against the people who believe the complete opposite of me as long as they are good people who don't hurt others or try to force their beliefs onto others. You can still love someone without agreeing with them on every issue. As long as you share similar core values, there can still be a healthy bond. Furthermore, I wish no harm on anyone who believes vaccines are good for them or genuinely believes what the people on TV or in school tell them. In a perfect society, we would be able to "trust the experts" to tell the truth. But as long as you don't impose your beliefs onto me, then I'm all for live and let live!)

Getting back to problems with my education...for instance, I was told by my professors that there was no such thing as heavy metal toxicity or candida "overgrowth." (I've since learned that an "overgrowth" isn't a mistake by the body nor is it an infection. I will clarify this later.) However, as I've since learned on my own, these were in fact real and true and contributed to my digestive and neurological issues. We were basically taught that the body messes up, attacks itself, gets attacked by "viruses" in all cases (as opposed to analyzing the poisonous and toxic inputs and lifestyle choices that are going into our bodies), and it's up to modern medicine to "fix" our God given divinely created bodies. We were also taught that genetics are one of the most important factors in illness, which I learned is not the case. Studies on epigenetics show that we can literally change our genes and which ones get expressed, and it is way more about our environment that we place our bodies in, rather than "bad genes." When it comes to health, a miniscule portion if anything comes down to our genetics. There are many other factors of actual value, so I think we should be largely steering away from genetics. And we were taught how to treat disease in a hospital setting with toxic chemicals (prescription medicine) rather than how to **manage wellness holistically**. I'm sure in class, if I would've mentioned chemtrails and GMO foods and the dangers of vaccines as well, I would've been ousted as a conspiracy theorist. Most professors didn't understand how much responsibility we have over our health. Most professors rarely mentioned the impact of our lifestyle choices, and it was always about treating the disease rather than treating the **whole person and all the inputs** that go into making that person dis-eased. We never discussed in class the importance of the mind body connection, or a belief in something greater than yourself. And many of them often claimed there was never a need to change your diet, move more, get outside in nature, detoxify, or anything else that's actually essential for your health. It was always just eat whatever you want, and then when you get sick be sure to take these medications. According to many of them, sickness was caused by genetics or viruses or bad luck. There was very minimal focus on actually taking control over your health through all the factors that I have since learned about. As I've said before, modern medicine can be extremely valuable and can save lives during emergency situations. However, outside of these emergency situations, we wouldn't actually need medications if we only understood our bodies better. Many people simply can't or won't take control of their health, and so they end up relying on these toxic medications to suppress the symptoms and to convince themselves that the medicines are making them healthy. Also, by taking control over one's health from a completely holistic standpoint, which includes emotional health—if we all valued things such as eating right, exercising, doing the inner work, and promoting detoxification in the body, maybe teenagers and adults wouldn't turn to drugs to "feel better."

Just about every super successful person will tell you that it was never about what they learned in the classroom but what they did on their own time. You always have to be your best advocate and learn what you are motivated to learn. I realized that once I started doing my own research when it came to holistic health, nutrition and fitness, and sports performance; I kept craving more of it. I wished that classes such as these would have been offered, rather than classes in those fields forcing a disempowering viewpoint onto us. This is not to say that a teacher can't inspire you about a topic or enrich your mind on topics you didn't even know existed, because there definitely are some amazing teachers out there. A select few of my teachers were inspiring and knowledgeable; they are just super rare and hard to find. My concern is with the people in charge of the system as a whole. I don't believe it's set up in peoples' best interests. It frustrated me that I would be so excited and inspired as soon as I would watch an interesting podcast, find an awesome YouTube video, or read an informative book, but then once I entered the classroom all of that motivation would evaporate. It was especially disheartening how by the time I entered high school, it was all about cramming information for the test and then blurting it out onto the paper, and forgetting it right after because there's always another exam coming up. No information will ever truly be retained that way. One thing that often made me different from others is that when I want to learn something I don't just want to hear the general. I want to ask as many questions as possible so I can know ALL ABOUT IT!

Take my physical therapist Andreas Saltas (aka @bodmechanic). He might be the smartest person I know when it comes to the human anatomy, understanding the function of every muscle, and how to help people heal from major injuries. Other doctors will tell you most of these injuries can't be fixed because that's what they were taught. They just treat the symptoms, not the root cause. But, Andreas didn't take no for an answer. If you ask him, school was pretty useless for him other than it gave him the title that he needed to get people to trust him. How is it that people who went to the same schools as he and acquired the same knowledge as he don't know 1/100th of what he does? Because he learned by researching himself, reading books, having mentors, and testing through trial and error. And today he is one of the most successful physical therapists/kinesiologists in the world. It doesn't matter how many years you went to school. Much of the time this just ties you deeper into the system and leaves you in more debt. As I said earlier, you need to be questioning everything you hear in school. And true learning most of the time won't be coming in the classroom unfortunately, based on the way the system is set up. There are countless other examples of successful people who didn't rely on school to be smart; they took what they were motivated and inspired to learn about and learned on their own. But, keep in mind those who didn't rely on school or didn't go to college or dropped out, did not just sit on their butts and become lazy. They got to work on their dreams. Once again, this doesn't apply to everyone. This is just my point of view and I'm not saying that school is always horrible for every single person, it's just not for everyone. Anyway, I did finish school for my parent's sake, but I always made sure that I was keeping my side hustle going and constantly learning new things on my own and getting out there and putting these things to use. There are a plethora of ways to learn these days, from podcasts, to YouTube, to books, to real life people with knowledge; it's all out there…you just have to be willing to seek out the information!

IT'S NICE TO BE NICE
Chapter 31

I always had the goal of being the nicest person and my friends and family often regard me as such, which is one of the best compliments I can receive. The way I was raised was to be the best person I could possibly be. As I got older I realized that doing good things for others has a positive chain reaction effect. Positive energy is contagious. Sometimes all it takes is a smile or a simple kind act to bring someone the positive outlook on life that he or she needs, and then it starts to have this ripple effect. I try to take this idea of creating positive chain reactions into my content as well. When you raise someone's spirits and vibrations, they can then take that into their next human interaction and make the next person feel good. Is there a better feeling than that? It's nice to be nice. And when you understand that we are all connected and how the law of one means we are all extensions of the one creator, you realize why it feels great to make others feel great. One day in 2017 I walked into the cafe at my gym, and the guy who was working the register that day says to me something along the lines of, "It's always so nice to see you Jared. You are always so happy and are such a hard worker, doing your workouts every day. It's so nice to see you always smiling." Now, I have been told by a lot of my friends and family and others in the past that I raise their spirits and they appreciate my positivity. But, this one really surprised me. I was extremely friendly whenever I would go to the cafe and sometimes would get into conversations with the workers. For instance, one worker with whom I was friendly would often comment on how I was always smiling and my strong work ethic, and I would tell him how I was so happy to see him too. However, I didn't really know this particular guy very well. We had never had too much interaction aside from some pleasantries, but my energy must have radiated to him and it was contagious. Also, keep in mind that I was still experiencing my speech challenges, and I was still going through a lot of tough stuff with my health. And truthfully, I wasn't always happy in spite of trying to portray that I was. But, others had been taking notice of my outlook on life and by seeing my smiles and my friendliness, this was enough to put a smile on his face and to give him positivity. I was truly taken aback and so thankful that he took notice of this because it made me feel better too. And I'll bet that the rest of the day and maybe overall he was a more positive person to be around, which put everyone who encountered him in a better state of mind as well. And it all started with a simple smile and just being my happy and friendly self. I didn't have to try hard to be someone that I'm not. I was just being me. If someone else had been through the health problems and life threatening illness that I had gone through, it's easy to see why they might have become more bitter and given up on experiencing the wonderful life around us, but not me. In spite of it all, I wasn't gonna let my circumstances bring me down!

(This surprises many people to this day, how I could be so happy seemingly all the time, even with all of the challenges I've faced and continue to face! They say that by looking at me and how positive and cheerful I am, they would never know anything that I've been through! I tell them it doesn't just happen by accident...happiness is based on our daily habits—from our routines, to the people and content we interact with, the music we listen to, movement we do, the food we eat etc. And while we can't be happy 1000% of the time, we do have control over many of these habits that actually contribute to more happiness!)

MY HEALTH ISSUES WEREN'T DONE WITH ME YET...THE HARDEST WAS YET TO COME

Chapter 32

After the summer of 2017, things really seemed to be going well. It seemed like my speech was progressing, my body was getting better, and I was injury free. I was jumping well and getting more athletic and stronger than ever. I thought I was in a pretty good place. I was happy with my friendships. Family was all good and well. I was almost done with school and as much as I didn't like it, I was gonna push through it for my parents' sake. Things definitely weren't perfect, but it just seemed like things were turning around and I was on my way to putting the health issues in the past. Unfortunately the way you look on the outside never reveals the full story of what's going on beneath the surface...as you'll soon learn. Going back to 2016, as I mentioned, that summer I was sick multiple times with coughs and sore throats and was once given an antibiotic for a "mysterious infection." There was also one month where I started having some digestive issues. For about two weeks I was constantly nauseous and had no appetite. I vomited a couple times, but then I tried removing lactose and some other foods from my diet in addition to taking a probiotic, and within a couple of days I felt much better. Little did I know this was only a warning of what was to come, and I was only masking the symptoms. So, onto October of 2017. One day after a workout I came home completely drained of energy. For the next few days it felt like I could barely move. I thought maybe I was dehydrated because that day I had gone in the hot tub and sauna. I took a few days off. Still, I felt pretty weak so I booked an appointment with Andreas. If anyone could figure out what was going on, he was the guy. He had a private chat with me, making sure I wasn't doing any drugs or drinking, which I assured him I definitely was not and I never have. So then, he asked about my diet. As I mentioned before, I was following a pretty strict paleo diet at this time in an effort to get rid of inflammation, get my body superhuman, and to hopefully heal the brain that was affected by the trauma which would ultimately restore my speech. I had been on the diet since the end of 2015. I was continuing to eat "healthy" as I had been since 2009, absolutely no junk food. But, recently I had cut my carbohydrates a bit more while noticing that some of these just didn't make me feel great. Andreas heard this, and understanding me and how hard I push my body, suggested that I add some carbs back into my diet, explaining to me how important carbs are for athletes. I couldn't argue with that. While I was there, I ran some sprints on the sprint treadmill and got an assessment from him. I followed his advice and got back to my training and felt mostly better.

Then, November came and hit me like another train. Just when I thought I was past it all, I was in for a whole lot more. It started off during a few days in school when I felt like foods weren't being properly broken down in my stomach. So I tried a mostly vegetarian diet for a few days to see if maybe this would help to lighten the load. Then, one night after dinner, I threw up everything. We thought this was possibly an ordinary food poisoning or a "stomach bug." So the next few days I went back to my normal diet, and a week later I threw up once again. I tried going to a simple diet for a couple days consisting of bread and crackers to hopefully settle things down. Soon after, I got sick with a bad cold and then came an episode with strep throat. (Also looking back I discovered that I had received yet another Gardasil vaccine in 2017, as per my schedule, because I still hadn't yet realized the harmful nature of these vaccines and their toxic ingredients. I wouldn't discover and make this connection until 2020. So once again this could've been another tipping point, even though as I will get into, there were many other factors as well.) I was really doing poorly, but I didn't see any connections. It just seemed like a bunch of isolated incidents. But as I learned, things rarely happen in isolation. You have to look for the root cause in every problem. Treating ONLY the symptoms will not get you anywhere. Soon after, I went back to eating normally and then went to babysit for a friend of mine. Prior to going, I ate a healthy dinner at Whole Foods where I had some sashimi, some paleo chocolate cups, and a healthy drink which contained some apple cider vinegar. That night I started feeling tons of acid building up and my stomach actually felt like there was a war going on. Thankfully, I kept things down when I was in front of the kids, but as soon as I left to go home I drove as fast as I could, needed to get to my parents and then to the bathroom. That night was awful. I was literally vomiting up acid and it felt like my stomach was going to explode. We knew that something was wrong but we weren't quite sure what it could be. I was constantly getting acid reflux and heartburn which, if you know what that is, it's one of the most unpleasant feelings, and I was getting it after every meal for the next year and a half. I was also in school during this time. So commuting every day on the train and sitting in class when my stomach felt awful made it extremely difficult to focus. But this wasn't all. Shortly after, new symptoms arrived. By December of 2017 I was stuttering and stammering with every sentence, oftentimes unable to say what I wanted, and sometimes my mouth would just freeze when I was trying to speak, or I would have to say "um" a bunch of times. This was on top of my already slurred speech (which had made improvements since 2014 as I spoke about). I always knew what I wanted to say, but something was going on with my brain where the messages wouldn't come out how I wanted them to. Then, came the balance issues. By April of 2018, I woke up one day looking at things in front of me and seeing them appearing tilted. It wasn't like I was falling over or anything, but I just wasn't seeing things the way I knew I should be. This was driving me crazy. So, I was in pain, couldn't even articulate my pain, things weren't looking right to me, and then I had my dad telling me this was all in my head and I was just stressed out, and my mom was telling me that I sounded fine and didn't notice my stammering and stuttering. I was crying so often and screaming and not understanding why I was dealing with this. And then to have no one believe me that what I was going through was real was possibly the most frustrating part of it all. I couldn't hold it together anymore. And even other family members and one of my friends thought I was making this stuff up, while others were trying to compare what I was going through to their own situations, which were obviously totally unrelated and just upset me more. Then came all of the doctors who didn't know what was happening. I went to my neurologist who had been seeing me periodically since my illness, and he assessed me and said everything was fine and he wouldn't worry about it. He offered me anti-anxiety pills and antidepressants, which I turned down, because I had done research and came to the understanding that these medications would just cover up the problem and not address the cause and would have severe side effects too (I have since done even more research and understand these pharmaceutical drugs to be toxic). I didn't want more meds, I just wanted someone to tell me what I was going through and understand that my pain was real and to give me a REAL solution. Then I saw an ENT who checked my ears to see if these were the cause of my balance issues. He didn't see anything wrong but suggested I get a brain MRI to find the cause of my speech issues. This scared the hell out of me. Then, I went to the allergist to see if I had any food allergies that were messing with my stomach. He didn't find anything. I went to 2 GI doctors for consultations and both said to just continue what I was doing with my diet changes. They suggested that there wasn't much else they could do for me. However, one suggested I take an antibiotic, Xifaxin. I was afraid to put yet another antibiotic into my system as I had begun researching the effects of these as well. I saw a neuro-ophthalmologist who also saw "nothing wrong." Also, by the summer of 2018, I had a brain MRI at the suggestion of my neurologist, which came back clean so that put me at a bit of ease, however left me more puzzled because I knew something was wrong. I was drawing the end of the line. This also only made my dad's theory intensify that what I was going through was in my head. But, even though there was yet to be a 'diagnosis' for what I was going through, I had 1000% certainty that I wasn't crazy. I was not making this up. I was going to have to be my own advocate and my own doctor. I would do my own research and find out what was going on. I did, however, find an ENT who discovered a weakness in one of my ears, and thought this could possibly explain the balance/vision issues. So, he sent me out to get some restorative balance therapy. I went there for a few months. The doctor was definitely a smart guy and the therapists were very nice, although he wasn't able to fix the problem as we still hadn't found the root cause. The problem was that nobody knew what was wrong and nobody was looking at my whole story or trying to see things from a holistic life perspective. And I kept thinking that if I let this problem continue without a solution, there's no way of knowing how bad this was going to get. At this point I was eating only two foods, steak and eggs, and even these foods were causing digestive symptoms! I started searching up natural solutions for my symptoms on YouTube. As I have learned, almost nothing happens in isolation; injuries, health issues, decisions—any problem stems from the root cause. That's what I needed to find. Something was connecting EVERY symptom I was feeling. **My body was obviously trying to send me a message—we just weren't speaking the same language yet.**

THE CONVENTIONAL WAY WASN'T WORKING

Chapter 33

Then, (still 2018) in my research I finally stumbled upon my first real possibility. It's a miracle that I even decided to click on the video. I was just sitting in my basement feeling lousy when I was searching through YouTube and almost didn't click on it, but one of the "ketogenic" people who I followed on Instagram had a suggested video appear on my feed about this thing called SIBO (small intestinal bacterial overgrowth). The video was titled "SIBO-My Gut Nightmare and How I Healed it." I watched the full 21 minute video and immediately thought this could be the answer to my problems. That night I didn't sleep again, but that was becoming more and more typical because of how awful my stomach was feeling. Finally, I thought maybe I had, if anything, a bit of insight. I showed my mom the video and she was in agreement. This girl had many similar digestive symptoms and other similarities, such as brain issues with unclear thinking and feeling depressed often. It turns out her dad was a naturopath and recommended a lot of natural supplements such as enzymes, oil of oregano, olive leaf extract, and a probiotic progression plan. They were also very nice and easily accessible. This may have helped to put a dent in treating some of my issues had I been able to meet with them or have a consultation. But after learning what I know now, it wouldn't have been nearly enough to heal me completely. At the time, however, I was pretty confident this was the way to go, in addition to my dietary restrictions. As I said earlier, with anything I do, I go all in. This includes my belief in it as well! I believe this is the best way for me to truly learn whether something is effective or not, and then during the process, determine what changes or alterations are needed. I figured if I did this for a couple months I would be feeling all better. I felt some small positive effects from the supplements, but the program wasn't comprehensive enough (for me) and didn't account for all of my health issues or the actual root cause of why my symptoms were there. I DMed the girl a couple times and emailed her father, and both were so nice and willing to help. However, I wasn't paying for constant coaching so I was unsure of correct dosages and what to expect. Also, my understanding of health wasn't what it is now. I was still in the early stages of my true awakening. Then, one day when I was at the gym, I started to feel dizzy, lightheaded, and nauseous. I had a horrible migraine with double vision as well. I felt really scared. We ran over to my pediatrician who said that I was experiencing an ocular migraine and that I needed more electrolytes and should start eating more carbs. This puzzled me because my body couldn't digest them. He prescribed me an antacid. I didn't want to take it, but my mom insisted. I threw up that night. Then, my mom spoke to the GI doctor, the same one who had told me to take the antibiotic Xifaxan in order to kill a possible bacterial overgrowth. But, modern and conventional medicine was not what I needed to fix the problem. As you'll see in a bit, modern medicine is what got my body into this mess (however, of course I'm thankful for Dr. Porter being there for my emergency situation and saving my life back in 2014). Nevertheless, with nowhere else to turn, I took the antibiotics for two weeks and made zero improvement, and even had another migraine episode a few days after beginning this course. I felt confused and frustrated again. It seemed like I was running in place and maybe taking steps backwards. I went back to certain supplements throughout the summer which might have helped a bit, but I still had not arrived at the root cause of the problem. I still consider this step to be a pivotal one in my journey. I fully believed that the symptoms had something to do with SIBO, but there had to be a lot more to it. At the end of the summer, I saw a new GI doctor in the city who we thought might have more knowledge and also offered SIBO testing. I visited the doctor around the time school was starting for my final semester of senior year. This guy was not on the same page as me and had no knowledge on any of the research that I had done involving natural healing. HE WAS NOT HEARING ME. He was totally bought into the medical establishment. The fact that he was not even looking for the root cause and didn't take my history into account made him difficult to trust. He basically told me that all of the research I had done on natural healing with supplements and collagen and apple cider vinegar and enzymes and probiotics was dangerous. (This doesn't mean that every "natural supplement" is necessarily good for you either as I have since learned and will go more in depth in a bit. I'm just trying to establish how we weren't on the same page with anything.) I still listened to what he had to say. After all, he did have some pretty great qualifications from some top schools and was highly rated. But as I said, life experience is the best teacher and will matter more than anything. Qualifications mean nothing if a lot of or basically all of the information you're studying is wrong, or heavily bought out and paid for by vested interests to support a certain narrative. And, as Victor (my naturopath/healing guide) often says, we are not data points, we are humans, so it is wrong to give everyone the same "treatment" and to try to fit everyone neatly into these categories. Even more, when doctors are not open and haven't even learned about every type of treatment or way of healing available in order to present them to the patient, this doesn't allow the patient to make an informed decision. I've learned to question all sides of a situation because one size does not fit all. "When all you have is a hammer, everything looks like a nail." He prescribed a potent antacid for me to take for a few months, but said that in 2-3 weeks I'd be able to eat everything and I would feel and sound all better too. He said that he knew this because he had "gone to school to learn this stuff." This was a classic case of his argument making an "appeal to authority," which is a type of "logical fallacy." As Alec Zeck often points out, many medical professionals use this. He also said that I didn't need to be tested for SIBO. The whole thing didn't make sense to me. Why would a natural body fluid such as stomach acid, which humans need to break down food and protein, be bad for me? Why would I turn off a bodily process with medication? Is he smarter than the human body? At first I would not take the meds but after a few more weeks with no progress, my parents insisted that I try them. We were running out of options at this point. I took the antacids for maybe a week and a half and felt worse than ever. They were not helping and were giving me new symptoms/side effects (which I knew was going to happen from my research). I was getting bad headaches and my digestion was worse than ever. No medication comes without side effects. Plus I knew that the research I had been doing on holistic health was correct—although not yet complete; I just didn't yet have all the information I needed, nor did I know of someone I could go to to educate me on how to heal naturally or possibly administer whatever treatment I might have needed. What was even more disappointing was when I went back to that GI doctor insisting on a SIBO test, he did one and said I tested negative and that there was actually nothing suggestive of SIBO. As you will go on to read,

I found out later that his method was useless as I most certainly did have SIBO—which although was technically just a symptom of the larger issues, it was part of my puzzle. And of course I was dealing with a host of other symptoms and health issues including digestive, speech and balance issues, as well as those which I haven't yet mentioned—toenail and foot issues, where I had to see a podiatrist at least once a month for a few years, to the point where they actually recommended surgery to correct my toenails. I never got the surgery, and incidentally now they are totally fine! I didn't care what this GI Doctor said though, he was wrong about everything else. I knew in my heart of hearts that my research was valid and on the right path. I just needed someone to complete it, figure out what was truly going on inside of me, and educate me on healing. I felt betrayed as I personally had experienced all of the wrong information taught from "top schooling." They didn't understand how to approach one's life from a holistic standpoint. In their minds it was all about prescribing people with medicine, and the only way to cure health issues was to lump them into a category and give them whatever pharmaceutical drug applied. This is not to say that all doctors are bad; some are fantastic and most truly are well intentioned. But unfortunately, college curriculum is so heavily influenced and funded by the pharmaceutical industry which ultimately profits every time a person gets sick. (In emergency situations, of course medications are likely to be used at your doctor's discretion and of course these doctors do save lives in those situations. Generally speaking we all should have the right to do what we believe is best for our own bodies.) Needless to say, practicing these symptom mitigating medicines (which in many cases don't even do that) while never addressing the root cause, will cause patients to enter a cycle of continually taking more medicine, only to get sicker. This doesn't mean that all holistic practitioners are great either, because sometimes even they are just focused on stopping the symptoms without addressing the root cause. **But, in my eyes, finding a great fit with a holistic health practitioner who truly understands the power of the body— including placing the body in the right environment while removing the obstacles to healing, as well as guiding you to understanding yourself and working in harmony with nature—is truly the only way to heal, as I would discover.**

172

Jared Weiss

STILL STUCK (RUNNING IN PLACE)
Chapter 34

I finished out yet another school year, which was incredibly difficult, feeling how I did. I just could not wait to get out of there. On top of that, I would sit through class while having severe heartburn and acid reflux no matter what I ate. I was also getting awful diarrhea and getting something called the runs. If you've ever had it you know that it is one of the most uncomfortable things ever. After doing a lot of research, I found something called a carnivore diet, so I switched over from keto to carnivore. I thought that what I was doing was fixing the problem, but in reality I was only mitigating the symptoms. I wasn't even intentionally eating "carnivore style diet" on purpose anymore, but in reality steak and eggs were the only foods that mostly agreed with me. And I soon discovered that only lean steaks worked, because I couldn't even digest fats properly. In addition, I was constantly nauseous and had no appetite. Clearly, I was not getting nearly enough vitamins and minerals that my body desperately needed. Furthermore, I was barely absorbing whatever nutrients I was getting from the steak and eggs. I tried this diet out for a few months and stuck it out, thinking that giving my digestive system a rest would clear up the issues. But once the school year was finished, my mom and I had to seek help from someone else since I was making no improvement. I thought maybe a naturopath or a dietician could help to solve these issues. During this time my speech difficulties were getting worse, and my visual issues were not improving either. It felt as if once again my whole life was crumbling right before me. As hard as I tried, my health wasn't showing signs of improvement. I was really scared and anxious that maybe this part of the life threatening illness would kill me or that I would end up back in the hospital.

Mom and I found a dietician in the city who was actually recommended to us by the last GI doctor. We went in with an open mind, and as soon as she started speaking, I knew we had at least found someone who was on the same wavelength as me. Finally, someone who was listening to me and understanding me. She told me how I most likely have a bacterial overgrowth and that my enzymes must be very low. After hearing my history with antibiotics and the intense stress that my body had been through, she was able to tell that I most likely had some serious underlying health issues that could be fixed if she connected me with a naturopath, whom both she and her father had used to solve their own health issues. Mom and I spoke this naturopath's assistant on the phone to send over a test kit, where I was to send over a urine sample and a saliva sample. Through electromagnetic testing, she would be able to tell me how well all of my organs were functioning and all of the health issues that my body was experiencing. I had to wait another month to get the results, and then a few weeks after that to get the plan and the supplements I needed to start the healing process. I had to stay the course and remain patient.

Midway through January of 2019, the test results arrived and revealed that I had a large amount of candida/yeast "overgrowth" as well as a small intestinal bacterial "overgrowth," (SIBO—as I had suspected), an ulcer, was suffering from leaky gut syndrome, and was not absorbing any vitamins and/or minerals. I would learn through my research that when issues such as leaky gut and candida overgrowth go untreated for too long, they can lead to cancer and other lifer serious life threatening illnesses It is interesting to note, I have learned that cancer is in fact a healing response by the body as a way of storing toxins that haven't been properly eliminated—it is not some random genetic issue—and it can be healed when you understand how the body works. (Cancer is of course an enormously complex issue, but this finding sheds light on the repercussions of toxic buildup.) As I'll get into in a bit, candida itself and the bacterial/yeast overgrowths aren't actually the ultimate issues—they are actually part of the body's healing responses and are symptoms that indicate that the body is dealing with the elevated toxicity. It makes sense considering how my body couldn't properly digest any food, thereby leaving my body and the cells malnourished. In addition, the test revealed that each one of my organs were not functioning properly. Basically all of my levels were not where they "should have been," and to sum it all up, my body was going through hell. And the most eye-opening part was that she was able to determine that what I was going through was a result of the large amount of antibiotics and steroids that had been used in the effort to "stabilize my condition" in 2014. *(As far as I knew at that time, they left a hole in my gut, poisoned my body, and essentially destroyed the terrain in my body. I would later learn about tons of toxins which include heavy metals, amongst other harmful inputs that were in my body as well. There was still much more I had yet to discover at this point. But, these toxins were not allowing my cells to function and detoxify the way they were supposed to. This naturopath found the presence of some of these toxins in the testing, but was not fully understanding of all of the causes behind them, the way the body works, and natural principles of healing. She was still operating from this place of the body needing to be "fixed," as she believed it to be "flawed." The problem was she was coming at things from a flawed premise as I would later learn and will explain in more detail soon).* Anyways, I did not know that this could happen, and I don't think any of my past doctors knew this either, unfortunately. She could assess my stress levels by analyzing the function of my adrenal glands and determine that my body had been through a ridiculous amount of harm, and that it needed a break and had to be healed immediately, or else worse things would ensue. She understood the trauma that I had been through and truly wanted to help me. This was the first time things were starting to make sense. Having said all that, this left me in a conflicted position as I realized that the initial misdiagnosis and modern medicine and harmful pharmaceuticals are what caused my condition to explode in the first place, yet was also required in the emergency situation to save my life. But ultimately natural healing was going to fix the problems caused by modern medicine. The conclusion that I came to is that modern medicine should be used for extreme emergency situations ONLY, which is actually what it was designed for, as Western medicine was developed during wartime. But it was then ultimately corrupted by Rockefeller and the pharmaceutical industry. Prevention, healing, and staying healthy should be done naturally and holistically by taking the person's whole life into account. I would learn more about the healing process in the coming years than I ever thought I could.

Once again, just as in 2014 when all this started, I thought this would be a fast recovery and I would be back to normal in no time. Once again, I was proven wrong and learned yet again that nothing worth having comes easy. The protocol was extensive to say the least. To anyone looking at everything I was taking, it must have appeared as if I was opening up a pharmacy. But, the difference was these were all natural remedies. I thought that maybe I would be adding back new foods each week, and noticing speech improvements regularly, but instead I was in for a long road ahead. The plan consisted of yeast killers, enzymes, and probiotics (in order to restore my gut microbiome, by giving it new bacteria to feed off of and allow it to break down foods easier), vitamins, homeopathic remedies, and methods to aid in elimination that could be done at home. The goal of this program as it was told to me was to first get rid of the candida "overgrowth" and then to build the gut and body up with probiotics and nutrients. However, as I've since learned, this was still looking at the body as if it was messing up, which is not the right way to go about it. Candida overgrowth, inflammation, leaky gut, ulcers etc. are all symptoms. They are efforts by your body to deal with its current influx of toxins and its state of disrepair. And if you don't make a change, you end up getting new symptoms, some of which could ultimately be fatal. Candida "overgrowth" is a symptom, not a cause. The body produces more candida to help it deal with the toxic heavy metal overload. In other words, they are indicative of bigger problems, but they themselves are not the problem. So to be clear, as I will go into more detail on in a bit, candida is actually necessary for our bodies. But of course, in the presence of heavy metals our bodies produce more of it, and this can lead to uncomfortable symptoms.

After two months I started adding back some vegetables that agreed somewhat with my digestion, but it was still only like 2 or 3. I was told that I had to go to the bathroom a certain amount of times daily due to all the supplements I was taking, which were killing the yeast in my body and moving everything into my bowels for elimination. I was speaking with my naturopath once per month unless there were problems, which at times I definitely did have. For instance, one hiccup I had was in the beginning when I was told to take a natural laxative because I was not going to the bathroom enough. After a few days, I was feeling awful, going to the bathroom like 50 times per day and noticing some nasty stuff going on. Something was not right. Thankfully, I stopped taking that and got back on track. With the addition of the new vegetables, I started making some tiny progress. I was still tired all the time, and was going to the bathroom to have a bowel movement an inordinate number of times per day, and it felt like I had to plan my days around my use of the bathroom. Every day was something new, and I was still constantly bloated, or the worst was dealing with the trapped gas seemingly on a nightly basis. A few more months went by, my speech still didn't show any improvement, my balance issues were still there, I was still incredibly fatigued often, and I was really frustrated. I just kept telling myself to trust the process. My best friends meant the world to me during this time and were essential members of my team, as you'll understand throughout the book. I couldn't even get through a sentence without stammering or stuttering, and some days I really just wouldn't feel like doing anything. I was doing my best to give my body whatever it needed to heal up and recover and was constantly doing research on foods to eat that would aid my healing process. I would also watch videos that offered advice to people going through similar symptoms. I retested a few more times and each time my numbers showed improvements, nothing that I could notice, but numbers that indicated that my body was healing and my organs were supposed to be functioning better—even though I've since learned that numbers don't tell the full story. For instance, by using synthetic vitamins in high amounts, the test results would give the appearance of one being fully nourished; however synthetic vitamins are not absorbed the same way as actually eating the foods containing vitamins in the correct proportions.

After the first 8 weeks, my ulcer was all better which meant that I could tolerate fats again. Yet, I hadn't been able to add any new foods after that first two month period. 6 months go by, and every time I tried new foods, nothing worked, as they would cause me more sleepless nights, more gas and more discomfort. So I stuck to my steaks, eggs, only cooking with ghee butter and coconut oil and olive oil, as well as the only vegetables that worked for me being spinach, sweet potato, butternut squash, and broccoli sprouts (not regular broccoli). Anything else and I would feel terrible. Even when sticking to that, nothing was perfect and I still had tons of issues, but those were what made me feel best in comparison. Going out for a meal was out of the question except for a plain organic hamburger at my favorite (and only) restaurant during this time, Burger Village (which still happens to be mine and James's go to spot!). James and Jacob were incredibly understanding and didn't mind only going there. James and I often had the same table with the same waitress who would always ask if we were brothers. Jacob would crack jokes at what I had to order every time, and we always laughed whenever the waitress would come knowing my order already. Jacob also found out that the chef always knew it was me when I placed my order of two plain organic grass fed burgers no bun nothing on it. James really felt bad that I couldn't enjoy all of the other foods and even ordered what I got a few times just so that I wouldn't feel alone. Then, when I would go to the Kass house for dinner, they were the best and so accommodating, making me steak with sweet potato and spinach, and always offering eggs and fruit or whatever else I could eat. It means a lot when you see people who truly care about you and want the best for you and go out of their way to make you feel better. Once in a blue moon if I went out with family, we would go to a steak restaurant and I would have a completely plain steak.

A year on the program goes by as we head into 2020. Recently, I had touched the 10 foot basketball rim for the first time and achieved a 36 inch vertical jump. I had become a better and stronger athlete than ever before, but I was still going through so many health issues that seemingly had no end in sight. I proved to everyone that you don't need situations to be perfect to do great things. During this whole time I was having countless sleepless nights. It was incredibly frustrating and upsetting. Some weeks I would have two or three nights without any sleep, even sometimes consecutively, due to all of the activity going on in my stomach. I still kept pushing along, doing my best to stay strong, making sure to continue hanging out with my friends, and trying to do the best I could on my athletic and gym goals. As I learned firsthand, it's not about getting what you want all the time, it's about loving and appreciating what you do have and making the most of it. And having strengths and abilities taken away made me appreciate them so much more once I got them back. It revealed hidden superpowers that I otherwise would not have discovered. My life was not easy; I was upset and depressed a lot. I felt lonely sometimes and alone in this fight, even though I knew I had the best support system out there. I felt like I was fighting against an unstoppable force. But, I always remembered where I started and appreciated the fact that I was even able to fight. Quitting was not an option. I knew I would find a way no matter how long it took.

FRUSTRATED AND MISUNDERSTOOD

Chapter 35

Many people didn't know the right things to say. Some would try to give me suggestions (as if I hadn't already explored every possible option). They would suggest that I see a speech therapist even after I just explained to them how I learned from the naturopath that my problems were being caused by issues going on which were connected to my whole body. These resulted in neurological symptoms; nothing was happening in isolation. Everyone has been indoctrinated to believe that symptoms are bad and you can take medication to get rid of each symptom or that some doctor can just magically make them disappear. In reality, symptoms are your body's way of speaking to you and telling you that something needs to be changed or that your body is trying to detoxify in order to heal itself. Some would insist I see a psychologist or another doctor even after I had explained how many I had seen. And I had made it clear that I knew what I was doing once I got to that point, so I was not looking for more people to tell me what was "wrong" with me and why I need to take x pill/medication in order to fix me. So few understood or would even make an effort to truly understand what I was going through as much as I tried to explain it. The truth is it frustrated me talking to a lot of people. They didn't get that I didn't want to hear their own comparisons to my situation. And I definitely didn't want to talk about petty things that don't matter. When I talk to people, I like being able to have real deep conversations. So many people just didn't get it, and some didn't even try as they were too caught up in themselves.

James and my mom, they got it. And it was incredible to see especially from James being so young with wisdom beyond his years. He would say things like, "I can't imagine what that pain must be like but I'm here for you." His whole family would truly show me that they cared about me and were supportive of what I was going through. And James would constantly encourage me by telling me he knows I can do it because I have overcome every other challenge. James is the type of person who will stand with you in the rain when he could be dry just so you don't feel alone. He would tell me that soon enough we'll be able to have a feast. He

180

always tried to reframe things in a more positive light for me, which is just what I needed.

My mom would talk with me for hours upon hours, as she was always the best listener. And I would say a million times, "When will I feel better? I'm doing everything it takes." And she gave me the encouragement I needed to keep going. My mom really is an unbelievable human being and she is the best mom in the world (as are both of my parents). I don't know anyone else who could deal with everything that my health put her through yet still continue to be there for me and my brothers and dad all the time. As anyone who has been through tough times knows, the best thing you can hear is first empathy—someone trying to understand what you are going through even though they might not fully comprehend it, they make the effort. And two, they tell you and show you that they are there for you. When you hear those two things, it makes you realize that that is an incredible person and they really are there for you no matter what, as they know you would do the same for them.

As I learned from my test results, the yeast/candida overgrowth was dead and had been removed from the bloodstream, but where did it all go and why was I not better? Although I had no explanation at the time, there were plenty of toxins in my body that hadn't been addressed by the current program, as well as other pieces of my life we still hadn't addressed. At the time though, we were still hyper focused on the yeast/candida overgrowth as being the problem. Regarding the yeast, it was supposed to go into my colon and small intestine and come out in my "excrement." I was told that this waste product was what was keeping me from feeling better and why I wasn't noticing more improvements. So, my naturopath recommended that I get professional colonics which were done at a place in New York City where I would go once per week. I was hopeful that one would do the trick, but no, it wasn't that simple. I did 8 straight weeks in the city, but I was still told to continue. Although it released a lot of toxic waste that needed to be eliminated and I believe this did have many positive benefits, it was still a mystery as to why I couldn't tolerate any new foods. I also learned of a castor oil treatment to help with detoxing the liver. And when I had stomach pain, I would lie down for an hour with a heating pad and castor oil on my stomach and it helped. I did this fairly often. She also recommended that I take epsom salt baths to further the detoxification process. These were all in fact great suggestions and helpful tools to incorporate, which my next practitioners would incorporate as well. "Whatever it takes" has always been my motto. Moreover, I had been making some good findings through my research on digestive health and natural healing, and I discovered a few more powerful "healing foods" to start incorporating. My body was still basically averse to any fibrous foods and any meat, except for steak, as well as a million other foods that I just couldn't tolerate. I was still sticking to my very limited diet of steak, eggs, some fruits, and sweet potato and spinach. But, I added beef gelatin, raw honey, collagen protein, raw milk yogurt, and raw cheese as those are some very good healing foods that my body could miraculously tolerate. These were definitely healthy additions, but something still was preventing me from fully healing. We found out about at-home colonics and after I did the first 20 or so, I was instructed to do 1 per day in addition to 1 epsom salt bath per day as well. I ended up doing over 50 colonics total, and although they are healthy and helpful for ridding toxins, they can also be very taxing on the body after a while and can dry out your insides and can impact your gut microbiome if you overuse them. When I realized that I still was not better yet, and at one point had to go like 5 sleepless nights due to my stomach feeling so off, I took a break from these and went back into the lab to do some more research. The current program was a step in the right direction and a piece of the puzzle, but it wasn't complete, and I still felt like I hadn't been shown how to heal myself, because that is ultimately where healing comes from. I hadn't been taught how to understand my body and what symptoms mean. But I was willing to learn.

Extraordinary challenges create extraordinary people, and I really wish the process of healing could've sped up, but the fact that I had to go through this for so long built up strength inside of me. All that patience I used would be needed to propel me towards accomplishing the rest of my goals. I would often say to my mom, "When will I just feel better?" Or "Why can't I just be normal?" I never wanted "normal" or "average" my whole life so I guess why start now? These challenging circumstances were preparing me for the extraordinary goals I had always planned out, and I was going to turn this pain into gains no matter what. I was gonna fight through it just as I always have.

LOOKING BACK, THIS WAS A PIECE OF THE PUZZLE BUT NOT THE WHOLE PICTURE

Chapter 36

Seeing some of the light through these initial practitioners opened the door to my questioning everything and wanting more, and it's possible that without this step I would not have discovered the healing I was ultimately seeking. As I said, everything happens for a reason. This first naturopath was not complete enough in her knowledge to guide me back to healing myself. I knew that I was on the right track, and I learned some new healthy tools and strategies, but we had still not arrived at the root cause as we were still in this attack mode rather than acknowledging the body's perfection. I had to find out why the body was doing what it was and help it along and be able to place it in the environment it desired for healing. I needed more. I needed to understand truly what was going on inside of me and what other changes and inputs I needed. She (this first naturopath) was perplexed as to why I was not better yet. I knew that natural healing was the answer. I just needed someone who understood that healing goes beyond the numbers and beyond just trying to correct the numbers or suppress the body's healing responses. I needed someone to understand that every single aspect of your life whether the foods, beliefs, detoxification, supplements, emotions, amount of sunlight, friendships, alignment with nature, sleep, movements etc. are either putting your body in an environment to heal or taking it further away.

By December of 2020 after having tried a seemingly random group of foods that gave me some severe anxiety and drove my stomach crazy, I made another discovery. I had been following this one YouTube channel for a while which seemed to have a lot of knowledge on the health issues I was going through. I realized that the guy I had been following had a course and a program of his own, and since I knew I needed more guidance and he had been right on with every food recommendation that had worked for me, I signed up for his coaching and his Facebook group. Due to a split between the group administrators, I will only mention the one whom I stayed with and the one who gained my trust. Victor

Jared Weiss

Cozzetto (owner of Vitagenics) is a wise traditions nutritionist, meaning he studied the Weston A. Price dietary principles and works with the Weston A. Price Foundation. He has done decades upon decades of research on essentially every health issue caused by the modern world, as well as every toxin and how to heal from their detrimental effects. And overall I would say he's true 'expert' in how to live more healthful lives in harmony with nature. After hearing my story, he had agreed that my problems were largely caused by the antibiotic and steroid treatment that I had been on from 2014-2015. However, the problems went beyond candida and leaky gut, etc. I was dealing with a heavy metal toxicity caused by vaccines, antibiotics, and steroids, as well as a poor overall internal terrain due to all of these harmful inputs. Keep in mind, he wasn't into the diagnoses, which I now fully understand why. All disease is caused by either malnutrition, poisoning/toxicity of all kinds, and emotional or physical trauma—and every disease is essentially extensions of those things (Victor likes to put them all under the heading of toxicity). So, he told me that if you don't remove these harmful inputs (whether chemically, physically, spiritually, emotionally), the body will never be able to heal itself. **As I will discuss in the following chapter, what I have learned is that your internal terrain will ultimately determine how you feel and whether your body experiences symptoms of disease. Symptoms aren't necessarily a bad thing, but they are how your body lets you know what's going on. It is your body's natural way of ridding itself of toxins, and if you are not taking measures to aid your body's detoxification pathways and to remove yourself from toxic environments, it will result in illness, especially in today's toxic world. Candida is produced in normal amounts in the body as a way to help you detox the liver and to account for large amounts of heavy metals. When the heavy metals don't get addressed, the body produces more candida and forms tough biofilms around them as a way of storing the toxins, so this is why just doing a "candida cleanse" won't be enough to solve the problem. It is not a mistake made by your body, however it is an indication that your body is trying to get rid of things such as heavy metals and other harmful inputs. Since your body doesn't make mistakes, it's up to you to discover why your body is having these symptoms and to**

185

find the root cause. This is why I believe my first naturopath program was not complete enough to heal me. It was focused on killing the candida, rather than finding out why there was so much there in the first place. This is the same reason why when the GI doctor gave me the antibiotic, it only made me feel worse once the candida grew back with a vengeance. These hard to reach toxins that were lodged throughout my brain and body and stuck to the walls of my digestive tract were causing all of my neurological symptoms, as well as my digestive issues. No one ever told me this in my college nutrition classes lol. Once again, my trust was required in order to heal. I started taking new earth based natural supplements that I had never heard of such as zeolite, bentonite clay, fulvic acid, MSM and greens juice to bind to these toxins and break up the biofilms that these toxins had formed. He was not focused on giving me a million different supplements and throwing them all at the wall to see which ones stick, as some natural health practitioners do these days. Each one had a designed purpose in helping the body and giving it whatever it couldn't get from nature or food alone. These supplements are found in nature to help the body heal itself through offloading of toxins. People and animals actually used to be exposed to and knew more about some of these items more instinctively for hundreds and maybe even a few thousand years in the past. I started eating and making foods such as kefir and meat stock from scratch. And soon I began making my own double fermented delicious kefir after having bought my own kefir grains from Millers Bio Farm, as well as long simmered bone broth which at first I couldn't tolerate. This was not just taking synthetic supplements to address nutrient deficiencies; this was about truly getting in touch with my nourishment and playing the most pivotal role in my own healing process. I began getting in touch with nature through grounding/earthing and getting out in the sun as much as I could. This is essential to healing. I was taking more healing/detox baths as well as trying out new forms of meditation. It wasn't a linear healing process, as progress rarely is. As Victor would often tell me, healing is not a destination, it's a lifelong journey. During the first few weeks I had a little scare. One day when I was supposed to go to James's house, all of a sudden I got really dizzy. Thankfully, after a lot of worry and frustration from my family, we got a chance to videochat with Victor who assured us that this was totally normal and it would pass. Within a few weeks after taking some detox support supplements and including some new habits regularly, I was able to get back to my workouts and some level of normalcy. However, trying to heal the 'incurable' was not easy, nor was it always the most comfortable. There were still a lot more sleepless nights and frustrating times and tears, but I forged ahead knowing that the truth in what I was doing resonated with me. This felt right, so I knew it was a matter of time. I wasn't sure how long, but there was no doubt in my mind I WOULD GET ALL BETTER and then evolve beyond that level. And the more Victor would educate me on my body's own wisdom and the more research I did, the more I understood what was going on. Victor was there for support every step of the way, as well as the other members of the support group on Facebook. And my best friends and family meant more to me than ever during this time as well. 10 months into working with Victor, I was able to add back chicken and avocado into my diet. Ironically James had actually predicted the year prior that we'd be able to have a chicken and avocado feast during November of 2021 and got it right as I was at his house enjoying this feast that month! Shortly after that I added back salmon, rice, broccoli, and brussel sprouts. I wasn't noticing massive changes on a day to day basis, but I was definitely beginning to see some huge signs of healing when I would look back and see how much progress I had made in a few months. Progress, when it comes to something such as healing the incurable or any of my other massive goals, doesn't happen in a linear fashion. In other words, you can be building the foundation and doing everything right for years, but 2 years later, seemingly out of nowhere you might notice a huge change that only happened because of the years where you kept at it! So, for me this meant that even though my ability to digest these foods was clearly improving, I was still needing to revolve my days around using the bathroom, my speech still wasn't really showing improvements, and my energy and sleep would be really good some weeks but then really bad others. I had to continue to trust God's timing and trust the process.

At this time (middle of 2022), even though I was confident in everything that I was doing with Victor, I felt that maybe I could use some updates or just an additional viewpoint to enhance my current program and keep me moving forward on my healing journey. I wasn't looking to change what I was doing, just enhance and update it based on where I had progressed. I also make it a point to never stop learning. Regardless of how much I think I know, there might be someone out there who knows something that I've never heard or just has a different perspective.

Cassie Huckaby-Adding another member to my healing team...

In August of 2022, I felt it was time to bring one more member onto my healing team to hopefully help take me across the finish line and to complete all of the knowledge I had been seeking. As you read about, I had definitely made really solid progress in the year and a half prior. I was definitely pleased with all of the knowledge I had acquired and the improvements I had made, and I tried my best to focus on these, as these were massive. However, I was feeling a bit discouraged as I was still feeling heavy, had low energy, and still couldn't go out of my house without worrying about needing the bathroom as my stomach was constantly active. And all of my speech issues were still present. So, in came Cassie. We realized that I had been on the heavier toxin binders (bentonite clay and activated charcoal) for a long time, and it was time to start backing away from them and to only use them when I needed them, as opposed to an everyday basis. I fully believe these were extremely pivotal early on for me in supporting detoxification—by helping me go through it more smoothly and getting me to a better place by giving the body less work to do, as well as helping my body properly digest and finally tolerate many new foods. However, as Cassie put it, with all of my digestive issues going on, it was as if my stomach was working from a debt standpoint in terms of energy that could be devoted to digestion. So, even though these tools were super helpful early on, to keep pulling from the gut—which can also pull some minerals too—for too long is very taxing. I learned that when it comes to using most binders, it is best to use them short term or for set periods of time, and to make sure the body is super nourished and hydrated during this time (although there are certain ones that can be used beneficially long term as well). I had actually suspected this for a while, and Victor had agreed. Victor was actually very much in line with all of the updates I was doing, which was comforting to know, as I trusted both practitioners and gained so much from each of them! Cassie helped me understand a deeper part of my personality as well, which is that I sometimes take a good thing and go too far. I even opened up and started crying as I told her that one of the main reasons why I just want to get better already is because I'm trying to inspire James and all these other kids and people in general! And I want them to believe that anything is possible by seeing my success. So, it hurt me every time to have to say that I'm not better yet but I'm getting there. As James had already told me, which was also very profound, he saw me as being all better, because he wasn't focusing on how far I still had to go. He was looking at all of the massive improvements I had already made. And I had done all these incredible things while going through these challenges. He said that if I get so caught up in being 100% better, I'm gonna be missing out on all of the amazing improvements I've already made as a result of my dedication and persistence. He suggested focusing on what I need, which is to get .1% better each day without stressing myself over needing to be at the end goal. Cassie reiterated this when she told me that anyone can believe in something once it's done, but it takes a special person like me to show people that I believe in the end result when I'm not there yet. She said that what I'm showing them is actually way more valuable than the finished product. Furthermore, she said she would rather me obsess over the things that make me happy and make me feel good rather than obsessing over every little nutrient or detail (even though I find those things make me happy too)—but I get where she was coming from as far as making sure I don't overdo anything. It's almost like in the *Uncle Drew* YouTube basketball series, when they talk about "mastering the fundamentals so you can forget them." She wanted me to take all this amazing and true knowledge I had and live it without needing to overthink it. She told me to take a truth and then let go of control, or in other words, let go of the outcome. She compared it to someone wanting to get a tan. If someone only has one day to do it, and they then go out in the sun all day, they're going to be ignoring natural laws and their body's cues to get out of the sun and will end up sunburnt. Sun is good, but overdoing sun isn't better. We then worked on incorporating certain other tools for detoxing. This was important based on where I was, even though as I said I fully believe what I was doing early on was necessary too! I began incorporating castor oil packs once again, and more epsom salt baths, and one of my favorite habits—saunas (which is where the best conversations always take place at my gym). She also made it clear that in order to get my body right, I needed to stop when I was feeling good, rather than push towards a deficit whether in my workouts, saunas, etc. She really wanted to try to get me to do whatever I could to get to sleep earlier. However, no matter how hard I tried, for months (and the years prior), my body just wasn't always able to do this. I believe this was one of those things where I had to complete more healing, and then my sleep would get better, rather than the other way around. In an ideal world, I would be able to follow every single suggestion perfectly and everything would go smoothly, however the body is gonna do what it's gotta do. This isn't always easy or comfortable, and it's important to be understanding of your situation. You can't force things to happen whenever you want it to all the time or stress about it; I learned that oftentimes you have to let up control for better results. She also suggested stuff similar to Andreas's recommendations, which was a cool coincidence—such as lymphatic massages which I really enjoyed and turned it into a relaxing practice while using a gua sha tool and different oils (Victor had recommended these too), as well as vision training, and the importance of turning on my parasympathetic nervous system because as my speech and digestive issues demonstrated, my body was constantly in this fight or flight state! This was all profound stuff and just what I needed to combine with everything that Victor had taught me to get me over the finish line. I was still having my bone broths, kefir, fulvic acid, teas, and coconut water of course, as well as keeping up many of the same habits, while also adding on new ones. She was totally in alignment with my belief that everything happens exactly when it's supposed to. She said how alike we are in how our final input that led to each of our health issues was actually the same vaccine, and how we were also both the best "tryers," and so it takes one to know one, and we are always striving to be the best which sometimes leads to us doing too much. I needed to trust God's timing more than ever, rather than force my control over the situation.

RECENT IMPROVEMENTS AND UPDATES AS A RESULT OF MY DEDICATION TO TRUSTING THE PROCESS

Recently, I noticed that I can have essentially any food now, and there aren't any particular foods that will trigger symptoms in any way! Although of course I still stick to my dietary and overall health principles and am choosing to be cautious, I am now at the point where I can be a bit more flexible and it won't negatively affect me! That's a long way from when I could only eat 2 different foods… Also, I have gotten to the point where I can take an occasional little break from using the tools, and I can still feel relatively fine (although the tools are of course still an essential help for my body and part of my routine). There was a period of time when going without the tools for even just a few days, the toxins would pile up, and I would feel horrible and could barely function due to nausea, stomach discomfort, and inability to sleep. Now, after having put all the work in with detoxing and understanding how my body reacts to everything, I know my body better and understand when I can take breaks here and there in order to make when I do use the tools even more effective! (Having said that, I've realized that for me, the reason why it can be challenging to take too long of a break is because since I've started loosening up the toxins and stored waste, I've essentially signaled to my body to start releasing more, so this way it can accomplish more healing. So I believe it's likely that until this part of the process is finished, I will have to do my best to balance everything out and continue helping my body along. I am definitely able to get away with longer breaks than I initially was, as I've learned how my body responds to everything, and since I've offloaded a ton already!)

Furthermore, my sleep has improved drastically as well! If you recall, there were periods of time when I would have several days in a row of no sleep! Now, generally speaking I can sleep through the night and get super high quality sleep. I'm still not able to do the idealistic "in bed before 10" thing, as I still fall asleep on the later side, but maybe that's just where my body is currently at or it is just based on my daily rhythms. I'm sleeping pretty comfortably for 7-9 hours just about every night, which I think is pretty amazing!

Now, although I was hoping to be "fully healed" by the time my book came out, I'm still not quite there just yet. My healing journey is continuing slowly but steadily. I still have my days where my body is either going through a lot of elimination or I feel it needs some extra help with detoxing, and this of course isn't always 100% comfortable or ideal when it comes to making plans. But on those days, I just have to support my body and give in however I can. I still have my occasional struggles, and I'm constantly adjusting as my body continues its healing process. No one ever said healing from a life-threatening illness was going to be easy. However, I understand this is a journey, and I'm here for all of it! I also see all the massive improvements I've made and realize the only way I got there was by taking it one day at a time, focusing on the daily tasks at hand, and adding up enough of the right inputs…but I do see the end of this phase and the light at the end of the tunnel coming soon! In order to get there I have to continue to have faith in trusting the process, and it will happen when it is meant to!

Due to my wealth of experience, I've also gotten really good at listening to my body. Even though there are plenty of great well intentioned suggestions that I've heard online and from my healing guides, above all, I've found the best results when listening to my own body and reacting accordingly to whatever responses it is telling me. The interesting piece is, once I had what I believe to be the best holistic health/natural healing practitioners on my team and received their help at the exact timing I needed their individual bits of knowledge, it was still up to me to use all this knowledge and make it mine. No matter how good what someone is telling you may sound, it's still up to you to find what resonates best with you and experiment for yourself, plus I had all of my own research to add in as well. I felt that now I had all the pieces of my puzzle, and now it was up to me to live my life in the best way that constituted healing for me. It was up to me to put my own spin on everything I had been taught and put it into practice! I needed to make my healing routine fully my own! Victor is still currently my main naturopath and the person to whom I look for guidance when it comes to anything health related, but he also empowers me with the knowledge I need in order to do what feels right for me. For instance, some of the more recent intuitive practices I started

192

incorporating into my healing approach have been intermittent fasting and enemas. The intermittent fasting where I've dropped down to 2 meals per day most days gives my digestive system a break, and most mornings I'm not even hungry early on, so this allows me to be more productive, and allows my body to focus on autophagy or regeneration of cells, as well as healing other areas of the body. The human body was not designed to always be digesting throughout all hours of the day. And the other practice which has been incredibly helpful, due to Victor's recommendation (as well as learning about the benefits of enemas from Dr. Steph Young), was doing MSM enemas. The body, when it's overburdened with toxins, needs some extra help in clearing these out and getting rid of what I discovered to be this mucoid plaque or sludge that builds up in the body. Especially when implementing all these other detoxing tools to aid the body, as I mentioned earlier when it came to the colonics, it is necessary for that waste to leave you, so this way nothing gets reabsorbed. Enemas have been an extremely helpful, almost essential addition to my protocol, however as with anything else I've done, it's pivotal to listen to my body and not overdo anything. I also recently reincorporated binders (activated charcoal in particular). After taking a short break, I still take PBX and PB zeolite (from Touchstone Essentials) just about every day along with Fulvic acid since those are all more gentle binders. However, after taking a long break from the heavier binders like the charcoal, I started to learn more about how each tool works on its own and went back to researching. I began experimenting, and something else clicked. The reason why every time I tried taking a break from the detoxing tools, I would feel so horrible, is because those tools were loosening up the toxins (which is what I wanted). But I didn't have something to gather up those toxins and move them all out of the system in a complete fashion. A post I saw summed it up well: "Trying to detox without binders is like sweeping without a dustbin." Of course every person is different, but now by knowing how to time each tool as well as knowing when to pull back and take breaks from certain tools, I have been able to successfully incorporate charcoal to "clean up" the loose toxins and make me a bit more comfortable. This also gives me the chance to take longer breaks from the heavy detoxing tools in a more comfortable way. Knowing how to loosen and remove the toxins was an essential first step, but knowing how to gather them up and remove them in a complete way seems to have been a missing ingredient and the missing piece to this massive puzzle!

I believe one of the most important points of my healing journey, especially from a mental/emotional/spiritual standpoint, was shortly after James had mentioned to me this idea of him already seeing me as all better. He had seen where I started from to how much I had progressed several years into my healing journey, even though there was still room to improve and my healing wasn't complete yet. After thinking about this, I realized what he was saying and I felt the same way. My speech issues did not limit me from doing anything I set out to do. I had my own podcast/YouTube channel, I was crushing it in the gym even though my health challenges/detoxing made it harder, I had the best friend in the world, the best family, I was meeting all these incredible people from my gym Lifetime Fitness who all loved talking to me, and I was writing this book. So, really as James said, "What's going to change when you're 'all better?'" Of course it's going to be an unbelievable accomplishment and it will make things easier, but I'm already doing everything I set out to do. Once I came to this realization, even though I knew I was never going to let these health issues limit me; once I had arrived at this amazing place where in spite of still going through these challenges, I knew that I was living my best life and that the speech issues and digestive issues were actually perfect for me during this time as a way of showing people what's possible, a huge load was lifted from me! Accepting what you can't change is different from settling for less. I wasn't stopping on my journey to overcoming these health issues, but I stopped seeing them as disorders and started seeing them as daily challenges that can be overcome every day. (That's also why I say I'm "healing" from health challenges rather than "suffering" from them.) Yes, were my heavy detoxing days sometimes getting in the way of my plans, or were my speech issues making it more of a challenge to get my message out to the world? Of course. But overall, in the big picture, these things did not stop me in the slightest. Daily challenges can be overcome whereas disorders are seeing things as wrong, and that can't be changed. It's like for the average person, they can just speak freely, but me I'm pushing a 10 lb weight every time I speak …that doesn't mean I can't still get my message across, and I have the evidence to back that up! Moreover, by doing the podcast and by having James and all of my gym friends/podcast guests reinforce to me that they valued what I was saying, no matter how long it took me to get it out, I began to become more confident in my speech as well. Of course some people who still couldn't understand my story weren't worth wasting my time on. But, I began to love myself with my stammering and stuttering or without. I began working on healing with a love for myself rather than this feeling of shame. Of course some days it was harder to see this than others, and I still had my challenges around people who didn't make me feel as comfortable being my true self, but this was a powerful shift in my perspective! Early on, I used to think that my story was only valuable once I got "all 100% better," but what I realized was that in so many ways I already was better, and I was showing everyone the process and all these amazing things I was already doing—so once the rest of my healing journey was complete, I'd actually be "beyond better!"

Another special pivotal point in my journey was actually finding Alec Zeck. Prior to finding out what I believe to be the truth on what actually causes disease and prior to finding out that no virus has ever been proven to exist (since no virus has ever truly been isolated and found to cause disease), I was convinced that my body had messed up. Every doctor had tried to convince me that my body was at fault for this random occurrence and basically that my body didn't operate correctly. And moreover, once further health issues ensued, I was basically told that it was all incurable and that was how I would live the rest of my life. The reason why I'm so vocal and feel the need to discuss these "controversial topics" is not for the sake of stirring up controversy. **It's because of how these lies directly affected me and how they tried to disempower me.** And by me having my eyes opened to these "hard truths" as I see them, I feel that I took back control over my situation, and this knowledge empowered me with realizing how special I and all humans are if we would only understand our potential and our ability to co-create our realities. This is not just reserved for a few of us, but all of us have this! With enough proper inputs and patience, I believe we can heal from anything and totally flip the script. Finding this whole world of holistic

195

health put me back in the driver's seat. I will address this point in even more depth at the end of the next chapter.

USING TOOLS/SUPPLEMENTS
Chapter 37

When it comes to supplements and/or holistic health tools, people in the allopathic community will try to convince you they have not been studied or are unscientific and dangerous. Even a few people in the holistic community will say that all supplements are the same as pharmaceuticals and it is all a scam with people trying to sell you things, while others live by them and only use them without any other lifestyle changes. It has been confusing studying the different views when it comes to supplements, but through my years of experience it is clear to me. Here's my take. One, not all tools/supplements are created equally, and there has to be a purpose when using them. Also, if they are trying to suppress the body's symptoms or to cover up flaws in the person's lifestyle, then chances are they won't actually help the body heal and are essentially being used for the same purpose as pharmaceuticals. However, living in this toxic world that we are in, I think it is absolutely pivotal to take advantage of the tools that nature has provided us with, and there are some incredible supplements out there that would have been found in nature by our ancestors as they knew of their powers (technically some of these aren't even considered "supplements," but for the sake of understanding my point, I will refer to them as such). Some of these would be bentonite clay, activated charcoal, fulvic acid, zeolite, MSM, castor oil packs, enemas, and Epsom salt baths--these tools can help the body stay nourished while helping the body to detoxify when used properly and in the right amounts. And I personally believe that when used correctly, these are totally in alignment with natural principles. I would never say that anything is impossible, however I don't know if it would've been possible for my body to heal from the severity of toxic damage had it not been for aiding the body's detoxification capabilities and using the tools mentioned previously (bentonite clay, zeolite, fulvic acid, MSM, activated charcoal, Epsom salt baths, castor oil packs, super greens juice, detox baths, Iteracare (energy healing device that uses the power of healing frequencies), enemas/colonics, etc.) These tools come from nature, and considering how our ancestors knew how to use many of these tools for thousands of years, I think it would be unwise to deny their essential role in my healing process. The right supplements and tools can most definitely expedite the healing process and enhance the quality of your life. I also believe everyone is different, so what works for one person might not work for someone else. Maybe some people out there do just need a few lifestyle tweaks to heal, but I believe others need a lot more help from these tools. The body is in fact always healing itself and always doing whatever it can to get better and keep you alive, and this is important to acknowledge. However when it becomes overwhelmed with toxins, it cannot detox as effectively, and that's where these severe health problems start. You can tell yourself that a strong mind can overcome anything as much as you want or ignore these toxins we're exposed to, but we do in fact have a physical body that can get overwhelmed and severely affected by these toxins. So, if you don't aid the body with compounds and tools that nature has given us, it can be super hard to fully heal or ever feel all better. Don't forget, I was at a point where I was only eating two different foods and was feeling pretty awful all the time in spite of trying to follow as many healthy habits as I could. I did actually attempt the route without them, and it didn't work for me. I'll reiterate, it's pretty challenging for the body to fully heal when it's being overwhelmed by toxins, whether under your control or by those coming from the environment, injections, and sprayed on us in the form of chemtrails, or sprayed on our foods in the form of pesticides, etc. every day. However, relying only on supplements and outsourcing your whole trust to them without changing and improving your lifestyle isn't good either. But, using all of the proper tools at your disposal to aid the body in trying to do its job is essential, along with every single input from your life. *Two, the body can only fully heal itself when placed in the right environment*. A lot of people forget that second part. Just about every person is not living in the most pristine environment these days! So, by not placing your body in the right environment and not giving it everything it needs, and not removing the obstacles to healing, you could actually be allowing the damage to continue. Lastly, an example I like to use is, if it takes 500 pushups to accomplish the same stimulus as 5 sets of bench press, why wouldn't you just use the tool at your disposal to be more efficient and get more work done? If it would take the body 20 years to heal itself without any help or supplements or anything outside the body whatsoever, but with taking advantage of all these amazing tools it will take 5 years, I think it makes more sense to use the tools. There is so much more that goes beyond supplements, as I've spoken about in depth, but when you pair them with an overall lifestyle that is on the side of life and healing, they are definitely an important piece of the puzzle and can optimize your life and can help you thrive! Remember that there are no magic pills though—it's all holistic!

Before learning how much power I had when it came to my health and the nature of reality as a whole, and prior to being put back in the driver's seat, every day felt as if I were being forced to sit in my neurologist's office to wait 6 hours for an "authority figure" to tell me what was wrong with me...and sure enough, I was told time and time again that my body had messed up and that I was attacked by some "deadly virus." Once I started finding research from people like Alec Zeck, which made me realize that my body had responded perfectly, I then realized how powerful I was, not in that it was my responsibility with what I went through because I didn't know about these things at the time, but rather it was within my power to go on my healing journey and to become better, stronger, and more resilient than ever before. And interestingly enough, that's why I love everything that I learn from going down the rabbit holes of many of these "conspiracy theories" or what I believe are "conspiracy truths." We were told from a young age to not listen to our perceptions when it comes to things like how we don't feel like we're moving, water can't curve and can't possibly stick to a spinning ball, etc., and we are told that power comes from authority rather than within as well as from God. So, by exploring these concepts, I actually strengthened my knowing of God, and it brought me closer to the divine and my purpose. We were taught in the school system about the "Big Bang Theory," as they wanted us to get away from belief in the creator. But once you realize that we aren't on a spinning ball and aren't seeing a sun that they claim is 93 million miles away, you then realize that God created our world and that we are here for a reason and all have a special purpose! We can co-create our realities with our free will that we've been blessed with, and we can understand how special we really are!

FINDING NATURE AND MY INNER SPIRITUALITY

Chapter 38

For a long time, as I had mentioned, it was go go go, and I was constantly working without ever taking the time to step back and appreciate the amazing world around me. Throughout my healing journey I started to become very spiritual and made the effort to align myself more with nature. I realized that we are all part of nature. And we as humans are so much more than just matter, and we are definitely not a waste of space. We are made up of 45-75% water, and that water consists of our thoughts, beliefs and emotions as evidenced in the book *The Hidden Messages in Water* by Masuro Emoto, as well as what we physically put into our bodies. What we tell ourselves, who we surround ourselves with, what content we watch, and how connected we are to nature will all influence how our lives turn out. And we can literally manifest our desires by aligning our thoughts and actions with what we want. It is incumbent upon us to use our free will to become the best versions of ourselves and level up daily. Nature is so beautiful—there is beauty in every step we take, every breath we breathe, and every human interaction we have. And what we resist will persist. Going by the law of attraction, it is so important to connect with what you want more of, as this will attract more of that in your life. And being connected with nature will promote more healing, love, and gratitude as these are what the universe runs on. Modern society has tried to disconnect us from our spiritual nature, but when you realize that everything is connected and that we are part of nature and we are one with the universe, you understand how this can't be neglected when it comes to anything you wish to accomplish. Sometimes, as I learned, you have to slow down, appreciate everything you have in the moment, and just be.

MY THEORIES AS TO WHY I GOT SO SICK...
Chapter 39

Some of the theories that I have developed in recent years as to why I got so sick are based on my research from my naturopaths, books, podcasts, personal experience, as well as my healing process. They are as follows... First off, I think it's possible and highly likely that childhood vaccines may have been the reason (or at least a contributing factor along with other environmental toxins) why I would get strep throat and ear infections all the time as a kid. This was confirmed by both Cassie and Victor. I have also learned this from some other prominent holistic health figures who I listen to as well. Also, growing up and all throughout high school, I would develop a severe cough during allergy seasons-it was so awful and would literally be non-stop. I couldn't sleep. My mom would give me ice pops all night to alleviate the coughing. I was given medicine for it that didn't help and these would last for a month each time. Now, it all makes sense to me. (Ever since going on my healing journey, this does not happen anymore!) This does not mean that everyone will have the same immediate reaction or even any "noticeable" reaction, however due to the toxic ingredients used in them, the negative reactions often manifest in other ways down the road that often get overlooked, and people think these symptoms just arise out of nowhere when really many of them are directly attributable to the vaccines. Many "experts" won't acknowledge this connection due to their years of schooling as well as the fear of being ousted from the medical community. Also, we all have different detoxing capabilities and different amounts of exposure to toxins, whether throughout our lives or even while in the womb. Our bodies are extremely resilient as well. This does not mean that these toxins are any less dangerous, but rather a testament to our body's ability to heal itself. My research shows that vaccines have toxic ingredients such as heavy metals-aluminum adjuvants, formaldehyde, and mercury (thimerosal) that don't belong in our bodies. As these toxins build up they are capable of causing a host of issues. And as the number of vaccines has increased, so has the rates of disease due to additional factors as well. *(If you want to understand where my research comes from on vaccines, some really informative books that I've read are "The Truth About Contagion" aka "The*

Contagion Myth" by Dr. Tom Cowan and "What Really Makes you Ill?" by Dawn Lester and David Parker, as well as studies done by Stefan Lanka. I have also learned a ton from podcasts such as Weston A. Price Foundation, and those done by Alec Zeck) So, getting back to my personal situation...as a result of the ear infections and numerous bouts with strep throat, I was on plenty of antibiotics growing up to treat these. Antibiotics, as well as any pharmaceutical drug, are filled with toxins that cause adverse reactions and inflammation in the body and don't allow for the body's natural detoxification system to form (while most think of this as your "immune system," I believe it is more of a detoxification system). As I learned from Victor, not only do these drugs/antibiotics poison your body, but they also impair your body's own detoxing capabilities. So, you see, it's all cyclical. A buildup of toxins can cause the body's need for illness, and antibiotics cause more toxin buildup leaving your body at a disadvantage to properly detox, which can impact the microbiome and cause malabsorption of nutrients—consequently disrupting the pathways of nourishing the body, causing an imbalance of hormones, cellular dehydration, decrease in organ function, adrenal cell stress, etc.—there is no limit to the amount of damage caused by this toxic overload. Next, on top of this, I had received the Gardasil vaccine/HPV just 1 week prior to starting college—a three dose series May 23rd, 2014-August 13th, 2014- and April 21st, 2017—I still had yet to learn about the dangers of vaccines. As I mentioned I wouldn't fully understand this until around 2019 or 2020. I, along with Victor and Cassie, all believe this played a massive role in my getting so sick—and interestingly, as I stated previously, Cassie had a similar reaction herself to this vaccine that led to years of health issues for her too!

I believe a good analogy could be looking at things like a bucket, and when you fill the toxic inputs in the bucket over the edge, they will spill over. Similarly, at a certain point, your body can't tolerate one more toxic input and is forced into severe disease as a way of trying to create a strong detoxification. In other words, did these added harmful inputs push me over the edge? I believe so, as do these other top natural healing guides/naturopaths who I've spoken to. However, it's rarely just one thing that causes such a downward spiraling of the body, even though

Jared Weiss

there are some "larger drops in the bucket…" It's rarely ONLY the last drop in the bucket. So, all throughout high school I had been sleep deprived and incredibly stressed out, overworked and overtrained. Adding to those toxins, it is also likely that the dorm building at Cornell I was living in contained a lot of mold (which indicates poor environmental conditions), as I've heard from one naturopath who knows that to be the case in that particular dorm. If you remember, even Dr. Porter (who's not into natural medicine), made it a point to say how possibly my body was exposed to foreign environmental toxins. So the environment in which my body was placed in may have been adding to my "bucket." Others in my building and the one next to mine had gotten sick (or also many of us had likely gotten these same shots prior to going to school and therefore, maybe many of us were sharing similar sickness/detox symptoms in addition to the potential environmental toxins and/or new stressors) around this time too. So likely, we were exposed to the same toxins (read Tom Cowan's books to understand why I don't believe it was some 'virus' or germ that caused my dis-ease).

The way I see it now, sickness is your body's way of trying to help you adapt to your environment. And being at "war" with illness will only create more dis-ease, as oftentimes "what you resist will persist" and will come back with a vengeance. Getting misdiagnosed (if you remember I was originally told I just had the flu) didn't help much either of course. Then, when you add on top of all that the fact that I was being pumped with 21 different antibiotics, multiple antiviral medications, placed on a ventilator and a feeding tube, was placed in a medically induced coma, and all of the medications associated with these procedures, in addition to the medication used to stop my involuntary movements, as well as given steroid and antacid treatment for the following 6 months… you have the perfect storm as to why I had a life threatening illness, as well as over 9 years of serious complications following, and the reason for my lengthy healing process.

Could it have been some super rare thing that caused me to react the way I did? Maybe…but based on what I know now, I have come to these conclusions and it makes sense to me. I feel that I've unraveled a lot of

the "mystery." Your body reacts to inputs and gives you outputs based on what it knows best, so there was definitely a reason why my body reacted the way it did. Bodies often have to purge toxins when they have been exposed to them for so long—they become embedded in cells, stick to the intestinal walls, and your body often forms biofilms as a way of setting them aside because it is unable to deal with them at that time. And if you do nothing to eliminate behaviors or toxins, they will continue to cause more issues and wreak havoc on your health. The germ is not the cause of illness as I used to believe. And we are exposed to so many toxins and harmful inputs these days whether through our food, glyphosate, chemtrails, 5G millimeter waves, heavy metals, perpetual fear, vaccines, toxic cleaning products, stress, mold, herbicides and pesticides, toxic water, overuse of antibiotics, overuse of pharmaceuticals, etc. (There is a full list of causes of illness put out by Alec Zeck). I believe that what researchers believe to be "viruses" are actually exosomes that help clean up debris in your body and help us upgrade to handle our new environment. And our body's terrain will determine whether or not our body can handle the upgrade. As Louis Pasteur acknowledged on his death bed after having debated with Antoine Bechamp on the issue…"It is not the germs we need to worry about. It is our inner terrain."
Furthermore, I have also learned through my research about terrain "theory" of illness and I definitely believe it to be true. This is basically the idea that illness is caused by what happens within your own body's internal terrain and whatever inputs are introduced to it, rather than germs and "viruses." We do know one thing for sure. People who live a holistic healthy lifestyle by taking care of their internal terrain doing things such as eating organic foods, improving the body's detoxification pathways, taking whatever high quality natural supplements they need, exercising and moving often, sleeping well, drinking clean structured water, avoiding toxic people, doing their best to avoid environmental toxins when possible (this doesn't mean overstressing or living in fear of these things, but rather being aware and empowering yourself over these things), keeping an incredible team of people around them, living with a purpose and believing in something greater than themselves, taking care of their emotional health, and meditating, are not likely

to have chronic debilitating illness and much more likely to live a happier life! And if you do "voluntary purges" (things such as enemas and other detoxing tools) as Dr. Steph Young refers to them as, chances are you likely won't experience acute illness as often or as severe as well. This doesn't mean you have to live absolutely "perfect" 1000% of the time. Our bodies are incredible and can adapt to just about anything, so stressing like crazy about every little "bad thing" out there won't be good for your health either. And it doesn't mean you should live in complete fear of the bad things out there and can never have any nonorganic food ever. I'm always going to try to do everything possible to live my healthiest, natural, close to perfect life lol because that's what I enjoy doing, as that's a part of me and I love myself so I want to give myself the best! I feel like some people out there talk about it like it's a chore to take care of yourself and take control of your health; when the way I see it is you GET to take care of the incredible body designed by God. It's important to recognize your responsibility and all of the factors that you do have control over when it comes to your health, as well as to empower yourself with every positive input, all while maintaining awareness and trying your best to avoid the negative ones as best as you can! Once again, it's not productive for your health to be overly fearful of the harmful inputs, just as it's also not productive to ignore them completely; but rather living a healthy lifestyle will give you the tools to empower you over them so that you don't have to be fearful.

As I always say, everything happens for a reason—without this experience, I wouldn't be the person I am today and might not have the perspective that gives me the utmost appreciation for living, helping, and inspiring others, and the proof that anything is possible! Maybe this also happened as a way for me to help wake others up to what's going on in the world and inspire true health and healing!

The reason why I wanted to include this part in the book, aside from the fact that I've become very passionate on the topic, is that we've been indoctrinated to believe that humans are vectors of disease. We've been taught that we lack what we need to be healthy, and therefore it's up to these big companies and/or governments to "save us." All this time, I was convinced that my body had messed up, and that made me feel really out of control and powerless for a while. It wasn't until I began studying and researching holistic health that I began to take back control and understood that my body didn't mess up, it was just reacting to all of the crazy inputs it was given. We've been taught that we are born imperfect and need certain injections in order to survive. I don't believe this to be true. I believe we were all made perfectly in the image of God, and any issues we have are due to our inputs, whether of our knowing or not. And when you don't know that something is harming you, it's not your fault. As soon as you become aware of this though, it is up to you to own it and make the necessary changes. We can overcome anything. I didn't really have any control over what happened to me, at least with the knowledge I had at the time, as all of these toxic exposures were out of my control and beyond my scope of knowledge as far as what it took to be healthy. I tried to be the healthiest I could, but I didn't know enough, yet I believe this happened to me for a reason. We have it all within our bodies and with the powers of nature to heal! We don't lack what it takes—we have more power than we could ever imagine. So, I believe this goes along with the theme of the book and can serve as a reminder to question everything you are told, don't let anyone put limits on you, and believe that you are special because you were meant to be here on this Earth at this time! Again, the reason for my book is not to start up controversy for the sake of starting up controversy, but rather to spread peace, love and positivity, and to help empower you to understand how amazing you truly are!

EVOLVING BEYOND "NO DAYS OFF"
Chapter 40

What I'm about to discuss only applies to those who need to be kept away from working because they're overdoing it, not those who are too lazy. It's the concept of pushing too hard and causing more harm than benefits to your body. As I mentioned earlier, I am one who takes things to the extreme and takes things literally. So, if you tell me no days off is what's needed to succeed, for me that means training hard 3 times per day no matter how little sleep I get and basically going until my body falls apart. This was my mindset for a while until I learned how unhealthy this was. Well this is what I have learned from my literal "No days off, no minutes off" mentality; it definitely was part of who I was and part of developing my rock solid mindset, because I was literally pushing day after day to the absolute limit and telling my body to keep going. As they say, "The road to hell is paved with good intentions." The real meaning of no days off is working smart and hard, and it means doing everything in your power to get better and to keep your eyes on the prize, but *giving yourself a break when necessary*. This also means having fun with friends and family because as I've learned, having fun has a tremendous positive impact on your work quality, and it's actually been scientifically proven that happiness improves recovery times and productivity greatly. Why do you think kids are able to run and jump for hours on end without tiring? Their minds are staying fresh and they aren't putting crazy amounts of pressure on every little action. In recent years, I have learned to balance both enjoying life in addition to adhering to my regimen. Being regimented is great but if you balance that out with enjoying life, you will get more benefits than you ever thought possible. It sounds weird or at least it did to me at first, because it took years of healing through a life threatening illness to understand these concepts. As recently as 2017 I was going to the gym 3 times per day, waking up at 4:30 am (2 weights workouts and 1 basketball workout), on minimal sleep (although I did take plenty of naps), with almost zero off days, while also going to school or working at camp. It wasn't until my health issues were full fledged that I realized I couldn't keep going like that. My body had forced me to make a change. It was keeping score and I couldn't ignore it anymore. It was time for me to start listening. I had been getting injured often and wasn't making the progress I wanted to on my goals, but I couldn't find the off switch. I had always believed that "more was better." But, I ultimately learned that some level of balance is necessary to truly be successful and happy.

I used to be the guy who had every hour of every day planned out and if life ever got in the way, my whole day was thrown off. I'd wake up super early to get a certain amount of shots up in basketball, then eat at scheduled times, workout with weights at a set time for a set length of time, and get home by a certain time so that I was able to get what I felt was enough sleep for the next day. That was my extreme mentality, but I realize now that I'm better off being more flexible so that I'm able to adapt when life hits. I am still very regimented, but I try to not beat myself up when something gets in the way!

I started to learn how if I am having a great time with a friend and we stay out 30 minutes past my "bedtime," it's not the end of the world. Sometimes having that great time is more important than sticking to my schedule. Of course sacrifices need to be made and there are times when you gotta cut your "chilling" short in order to have the most success. But, life is all about making the most of your experiences—you won't get that time back with that friend, so you have to be able to discern when it's worth it. Or if I have it written down that I'm supposed to jump train today, and I wake up that day after an awful night of sleep and my body is feeling horrible, truthfully I'm not gonna get anything out of that workout, except maybe a larger chance of injury and frustration when I don't jump well. I used to be the one who pushed through anyway, but now I understand the importance of listening to my body. Our bodies need certain things to thrive, so make sure you are giving your body these things. Life hits everyone in one way or another so if you break down when it hits, you're never gonna get anywhere. Create a schedule/regimen and try to stick to it but have gaps in there for when good things in life come your way. Eyes on the prize, but make room for happy times and exceptions because you don't get those times back.

"GOOD VIBRATIONS"

(Ironic title—because everyone tells me I look like Marky Mark aka Mark Wahlberg lol)

Chapter 41

Throughout my whole healing journey, I realized the power of songs in increasing my positivity and good vibrations (literally). Remember that we are all made up of energy. Be aware of all bits of information and energy that your body is absorbing, and make sure that the energy is contributing positively to your wellbeing. Music/sounds are part of your daily inputs. One song I love is "Best Day of My Life" by American Authors. I think it's so important to get your day started thinking and believing this could be the best day. In spite of the years it took for me to heal, I still would wake up every day believing this could be the day that I felt all better. And I would tell myself that even if I didn't feel all better, it didn't mean that I couldn't still make today the best day yet because I still possessed everything within me to make that happen. This is one of the reasons why I was able to have so many incredible times and experiences even while in the midst of my health problems. Because I wouldn't allow it to totally bring me down. I was going to make the best of it and I wouldn't let my circumstances dictate the outcome. That's a big mistake a lot of people make. And I have been guilty of this at times myself. We think that when we acquire this thing or when we finally achieve that goal or arrive at that place in our life, then and only then will we be happy. We don't enjoy the ride and appreciate the journey enough. If we can still have fun and thrive when things aren't going the best, then this can reveal true inner strength. If I would've waited until my speech was all better to hang out with my friends, or if I would've waited until my body felt amazing to do my dunk training or start up my YouTube channel/social media, I would've missed out on a lot. Often, when we do arrive at our goals, the feeling of pleasure is short lived. But, if we appreciate the journey and find beauty in the struggle of going through the ups and downs, then when we do reach our goal, we can say that it was truly a fulfilling journey as a whole, not just the last step. The other song I wanted to reference that I have listened to often is "The Fighter" by Gym Class Heroes. This song feels like my anthem and has helped me to stay in the fight and remember that every time I fall, it's only making my chin strong. And it reminds me that when people hear about my story, I want them to look at me and say, "There goes a fighter."

"Until the referee rings the bell, until both your eyes start to swell… Give 'em hell, turn their heads, gonna live life till we're dead, give me scars, give me pain, then they'll say to me, there goes a fighter."

I get the chills whenever I hear those words vibrating through my body.

THROW OUT THE RULEBOOK!
Chapter 42

There is no rulebook for how you need to live your life, so live it YOUR BEST WAY. You don't have to have your life figured out by a certain age, you don't have to be married or be in a relationship by a certain age, you don't need to be a certain age to have become a pro at whatever skill you are trying to master. At the time of writing this book, I have never been in a serious relationship, and to be honest I really don't want one right now nor am I ready for one anytime soon. Who says that's wrong? Maybe in a year, or a few years, or 10 years from now I will want a serious girlfriend and maybe I will meet the right girl for me who can enhance my life even more and whom I want to grow with…but right now I'm happily single, love working on myself and the relationship I have with myself, and I enjoy that freedom of not being tied down to anyone, and there's nothing wrong with that either way. There are plenty of married people with big families who are happy, but there are also plenty of single people who are happy as well. Do things when and if they are right for you and your purpose, not because everyone else is doing it! When it comes to school, who says you have to finish by a certain age or who says you even have to go to college or grad school at all? When it took me over 10 years of training to accomplish my dream of dunking, who said I had to give up? Others may have chosen a new goal or decided to do something else, but this was what I wanted to do and I knew it was possible, so I wasn't giving up on it. When I was grinding away at my social media, producing every day, and some posts were getting less than 5 likes, should I have taken a different path? And whenever people told me what I should do with my life and tried to detract me from chasing my dreams, there was no rule that said I had to listen. People who rush into things based on what others tell them they should be doing often end up upset and on the wrong path. Lastly, when it took me over 9 years to fully get better from my health issues, should I have given up and just accepted the fact that I wasn't going to get better and that it wasn't possible for me to heal? There is no timeline saying you must do something by a certain age or if you aren't doing this by that age, you must give up. Live life on your own terms and watch how much more you can accomplish. Trust

God and the universe's timing! I still don't have it all figured out. I don't know exactly where my life will go, and I can only tell you what I have learned and am still learning. Sometimes, when you have a dream that won't be achieved right away, you may need to have a side hustle that affords you the ability to work on your big dreams. For instance, while I am working on all of my massive dreams, I am also making money by helping out my dad with his work. In addition, I have also done plenty of babysitting and sports training and occasional nutrition and holistic health consultations. I am careful with how I spend my money. My side hustle allows me the time I need to build towards all of my wildest dreams. And of course over the years, all of the money that I had saved up between these ventures, as well as being a camp counselor for many years, has afforded me the money to spend on all of my camera equipment and the money I needed to invest and reinvest into my content creation.

Ultimately, remember that you can set your own standards, so you can shape this life however suits you best!

WHAT MY FRIENDS MEAN TO ME
Chapter 43

I used to hear the quote, "Friends are the family that you choose," but I never really knew what that meant. I just thought there was my family and then there were these people who I enjoyed hanging out with on the side, almost as an addition or a bonus. I don't think I really ever understood what the true meaning of a friend was until I went through the hardest times in my life. I have come to learn that family is not just your blood relatives, but those who love you unconditionally. If you ask the people I'm close with, they would say that I love to talk and love to open up and would probably classify me as a people person. But, in reality I'm a particular people person. I talk a lot and am an open book to those who I feel most comfortable around. Throughout my childhood, I had some great friends along the way or people who I thought were my friends. As I moved into high school, I felt I was the same kind hearted person as always, but my friends had changed. I began spending a lot of time alone. I was (and still am) very independent and didn't like going to parties. Furthermore, I didn't like hanging out in groups nor did I have a set group, so unfortunately this made it difficult to have friends. A relatable quote that I saw on Instagram by someone named Zach Tyler said, "Looking back I wasn't bad at making friends. I was good at avoiding the wrong ones." It's not that these people were all bad. A select few were very nice although it was rare to find someone who I truly vibed with. Every once in a while I would be invited to join them, but for the most part I didn't feel comfortable being my true self when I was around them. There was even a short period of time where I sort of thought that maybe I was just going to be a bit of a loner and maybe this was how it was meant to be and that I could be successful and happy on my own. I wasn't unhappy and I always carried around my optimistic outlook, but at the same time I wished I could have had some real friends who I could grow with and count on, because I knew how good of a friend I was capable of being and knew I had a lot of love and support to give. We all have a desire to love and to be loved. And I came to realize that we all need people in our lives, and it just takes sifting through the wrong ones in order to find the right ones.

If you are alone, it does not mean you need to stay that way, it just means you haven't found the right people to surround yourself with yet. And it's important to not settle for toxic people; in that case it is better to be by yourself. Too many people would rather be in toxic relationships and toxic friendships for fear of being alone. That's why I never bought into the whole "finding your other half" stuff. Because this implies that without someone else you can't be whole, which is a lie. The best relationships or even friendships come when you have 2 whole people who can build with each other and enhance each other's lives, not 2 halves who rely on the other to fill the void that they actually need to fill by first loving themselves! That's why getting comfortable being alone is a great skill to have. Because this way you never have to settle for anyone who makes you feel less than your best. And your relationship with yourself will always be the most important one you have. How do you expect other people to love you if you don't love yourself? You don't need tons and tons of friends to be happy—one or two really incredible ones, and anything else is a bonus.

When I did ultimately find my best friends, I knew that these were the type of people I had been looking for. But, it took until after the life threatening illness to strengthen our bonds beyond anything that could ever be broken. I realized that some of my biggest motivation to pull myself out of the dirt was knowing that I had to get back to see James and Jacob the next summer. James found out about what I had been through at a bus counselor meeting because his mom Jen drove one of the camp buses. I walked up to James that day, in my mind knowing everything that I overcame and how I had worked tooth and nail to get back to camp that summer. As soon as I started speaking I could see the concern on his face, yet I knew that nothing had changed and he made that clear to me. Jacob found out about my illness from a friend at school and texted me constantly to check on how I was doing, in addition to hanging out with me and encouraging me once he got home. Throughout that summer, my camp friends got me through the rough spots, as well as some of my toughest challenges in the years ahead. This was the true meaning of friendship-- friends who were like family. We all go through difficulties in our lives, some harder than others, and we sometimes feel like the valley just keeps getting deeper and it feels impossible to pull ourselves up. We also go through times when everything seems to fall into place perfectly and we succeed at our goals. Knowing that we will have friends who can help us pick ourselves up out of those deep valleys and rise to even greater peaks, while cheering us on, is what makes friends so important.

Just as with everything else, you have to work at being a friend and at being a good person. Being a good friend doesn't mean using someone. It doesn't mean having someone to complain to about petty things or to use as a punching bag. A true friend is someone who you can have real deep talks with. And something that I value so much is being a great listener. It is very rare to find that in this day and age. People are so consumed with what's going on on their phones or what everyone else is doing, but a real friend will make you feel like you are the only one who matters when you are with them. Maybe that's why I never liked large playdates and having tons of friends, because then you have to divide your attention and you don't get to feel the love as much yourself. And you have got to let your friends know how much they mean to you and show it too. That is what creates lasting, meaningful friendships and a few friends who become family.

Some people out there are so shallow that they will only be friends with you if you have a certain amount of followers, get certain test scores, have a large amount of money, or score a certain number of points per game. This translates into the conditional kind of friendship. These people have it completely backwards and should be avoided at all costs. The people you want in your life are ones who will love you whether you don't score at all or average 30 points per game; they will treat you exactly the same when you have it all or have absolutely nothing. If you are a great friend, your friends will know you and understand who you are on the inside. You will always support your friends no matter what, but it is also important to hold each other accountable when one of you is not living up to the high standards. Character is what matters when judging people. Period.

YOU HAVE TO SIFT THROUGH A LOT OF PEBBLES TO FIND THE GOLD
Chapter 44

I have had a lot of talks about this topic in my life. I'll talk about it with my parents or James and his family. The topic is how there are a lot of people out there who just aren't right for you. I'm not saying this to be negative, but to emphasize the importance of sifting through people to find ones who are worth your time. It's your job to seek out the best people for you. It's also so important to vibrate your own energy at a high frequency and so positively that you attract these people into your life. There has been a lot of research on this topic, and it's been shown that we all vibrate at different frequencies. Even the words you speak resonate differently in your body as evidenced through muscle tests, so the more positively you speak and think, the stronger your muscles will test. If you are positive and doing good things, you will be vibrating at a higher frequency. The law of attraction says that like attracts like, so if you are a good person you will find others just like you, because they will be attracted to you and you will be attracted to them. I have noticed that I am very adept at feeling the vibes that people emit in large part because I am a highly sensitive person. Oftentimes if I am around someone and feel off in some way usually it means that person isn't for me. However, when I meet or hang out with someone who is giving off great and positive vibes, I'll notice it and see how amazing I feel when around them. My body definitely knows what's best for it. Throughout my life and the schools I went to and sports teams I played on, there were a lot of people with whom I just couldn't connect. Many were not loyal friends and would soon ditch me or not talk to me because they would rather be with the "popular" group, or maybe I wasn't cool enough for them. When I would play sports with them, they would sooner put me down to make themselves look better rather than encourage me. I had to deal with a lot of these people as I'm sure that most of you readers can relate. And when I got sick, I really saw others' true colors. Some would avoid me or just weren't there for me. Others came to my rescue and were truly there for me, and I can never ever forget who was there for me when I needed it

216

most. Unfortunately, some people like it when you're down and as soon as you start the comeback, they start rooting for you to fail. And just as I have needed others to get me through the most difficult times in my life, I always try to do the same for others. I always believe in others, sometimes more than they believe in themselves. I have this instinct whenever I see people becoming self-deprecating; I immediately tell them they can do whatever it is they think they can't. I believe all of us are able to achieve far more than we think we can, and sometimes it takes someone else believing in you to show you that it's possible. One funny example of this in action was when Brandon (my younger brother) was little, maybe around 5 or 6 years old, we used to play basketball on this mini hoop and I could dunk on it, but at the time he was much shorter than me. I saw something in him that made me believe he could dunk on the hoop before he believed it was possible. I kept telling him to try again and again. Then finally he dunks it, but he holds onto the hoop and it falls on him. Thankfully, he didn't get too hurt, but I was really proud of him— even though I'm not too sure how thrilled he was with me at that moment.

When you are trying to form your inner circle, you want to make sure your inner circle is a winner circle. Typically, if your gut tells you something isn't right when you are around certain people, it knows what it's talking about. Be aware of people, even sometimes the ones who are close to you, who can suck the life out of you. You want people that brighten your day and bring you happiness.

Alone time can be great, and I love and value my alone time. I know that I can always rely on myself to be my own friend when I need it. But, as I also learned, being alone for too long can sometimes lead to negative feelings and depression. We need others in our lives, but they have to be the right ones. Don't get rid of all people in your lives, get rid of the toxic ones. Keep the ones who want you to succeed as much as you want to succeed and who make you feel happy to be alive. Equally important is being as encouraging for them to succeed as well as bringing them happiness. In the years I spent recovering from my health issues, I truly realized the need for family and friends who became my family. I

217

wouldn't be where I am today without them. Yes, it took a whole lot of sifting and getting rid of the negative bunch, but it was worth it to discover some of the best people in my life.

It is true when they say that you are the sum of your friends or the average of the 5 people who you spend the most time around. If you are surrounded by highly motivated people, chances are you will be highly motivated. If your friends are all genuine and caring people who are fun to be around and can display high levels of empathy, you will be capable of doing the same. Change your circle, change your life. As I like to say, "My circle's tighter than a cheerio," and I'll choose quality over quantity any day.

GET RID OF THE FLUFF AND THE TOXIC
Chapter 45

One rough part of life is seeing people who you think are your friends but will talk bad about you behind your back or to your face, or won't want to be seen with you when there are others around. I have no room for fake friends. Like Drake's song "Fake Love" says, "I've got fake people showing fake love to me straight up to my face." There are a lot of fake people out there, and they give a lot of fake love to use you for their own benefits. Some people are really needy and want you to be there for them when they aren't there for you. A friendship should never be a one-way street. It shouldn't be a stressful job; it's supposed to be flowing and you should bring out the best in each other. And another indicator of someone who is fake is when the person acts nicer in front of your parents than they are to you and acts like a big shot when peers are around. What you do with people like that is in your mind, thank them for what they did for you in the past and realize that they aren't there for you now and can't handle being a good friend to the awesome person you are. And if they aren't going to treat you the way you deserve to be treated, then you have to do what's best for you, and say this just isn't working out anymore, almost how you would end a romantic relationship. (Seinfeld did an episode on this called "Male Unbonding" lol). The best friends don't need to put on a facade; by being themselves, they are always exuding their best qualities. It's not easy getting rid of people in your life but it is a necessary thing to learn to do. It's also pivotal to let go of any hostility towards those who've wronged you in life, because that just drains you from moving forward. "Don't let anyone rent a space in your head, unless they are a good tenant." Why should you be around people who don't make you feel like you are incredible and realize how awesome a person you are to be with? Value yourself, value your time, and get rid of the fluff. Having fake people around is like fluff—it doesn't need to be there, and it's only adding weight that's making it harder for you to get around. Sadly a lot of people change for the worse as they get older, or maybe they were always like that deep down. But sometimes you are the one who changes and grows, and you outgrow those people because you are leveling up, and they want to stay where they are. Indeed, oftentimes a

219

friendship can take a detour when friends are going through different experiences in their lives—so you might go a long time without speaking while knowing the bond will always be there–and then somewhere down the road you reconnect. While other times, some people become jerks, and oftentimes you realize you spent years around that person. That doesn't mean you need to continue being around them. But this also makes you appreciate the amazing people in your life so much more. "Don't cling to a mistake just because you spent a long time making it." Get rid of toxic people and you will feel much better.

"THE LONELIEST PEOPLE ARE THE KINDEST. THE SADDEST PEOPLE SMILE THE BRIGHTEST. THE MOST DAMAGED PEOPLE ARE THE WISEST. ALL BECAUSE THEY DO NOT WISH TO SEE OTHERS SUFFER THE WAY THEY DO.".

ANONYMOUS

Chapter 46

One of the most amazing compliments that I get often and truly appreciate is when others tell me that I am the nicest person or nicest friend they know. I always aim to be that to people. Why not be the nicest and try to spread the love inside of you? I have been through a lot. I have cried a lot, experienced a lot of sadness and disappointment and anxiety, and have gone through a whole lot of things that others will never know about or understand. But, I feel like this is part of what makes me so nice. I know what it feels like to have no one believing in you, I know what it feels like to be lonely, I know what it feels like when life is weighing on you and it feels like things may never get better. The nicest people are often the ones who are the most understanding and can show the most empathy. I have become incredibly perceptive of how others are feeling. I can tell when they are sad or uncomfortable and when they need some help. I try to be the bright light in people's lives. I don't want others, especially my loved ones to experience the pain that I have felt at times (though I now see that the pain only made me stronger!). I want to take the burden so they don't have to. I always felt like I was given this amazing heart full of positivity and love, and I want to spread it to whomever needs it. Things may not always be easy. There will be disappointments, and anxiety and depression for some, and times when your obstacles are clouding the light—but it helps when you have someone tell you that everything is gonna be okay.

THE LONE WOLF
Chapter 47

Being a lone wolf can be essential at different points in your life. As I spoke about, you have to sift through the "bad" people before you arrive at the best ones. And you shouldn't settle for anything less. If the only people around you aren't in alignment with who you want to be, then you should not associate with them. I never wanted to change who I was to please others. I'm not someone who likes to compromise. To be clear, I'm not talking about having the same exact opinions on everything—if everybody thought alike, wouldn't that be boring? I'm simply talking about remaining true to yourself. We all try to have friends and have social acceptance, but when it comes at the expense of us becoming someone we're not, then it's not worth it. I am who I am, and if you can't accept that, then it's your loss. Others used to try to convince me to drink and smoke with them, and I always said no, and they couldn't understand why. It was easy for me. I don't want to do things that don't align with my principles, and doing those things wasn't going to help me achieve my goals in life. I'm not telling you what to do because that's your choice and I won't judge you for it, and that doesn't mean we can't still be friends, but I'm not gonna do it just because you want me to. My goals are much bigger than seeing how drunk I can get every weekend or being popular. I kept telling myself one day all my work is gonna add up and I'm gonna go farther than everyone who wasn't making these "sacrifices." Greatness takes time, and I'm willing to put in as much as it takes. There were times when I felt left out, but I would be my own best company, plus I could always count on my unbelievable family. And soon enough I would find my best friends in the world. All it takes is one amazing friend because one amazing one is worth infinite bad ones. So choose with whom you surround yourself wisely, and never be anything but yourself.

This is so important for a host of reasons. It sounds cliché that people are always saying, "Be yourself," but often they don't really mean it—however, it is a meaningful phrase. Be yourself 100%, do what makes you happy and eventually, as long as you continue to put yourself out there you will attract others who are the same way. The easiest way to see who

222

your real friends are is to see who's still around when you have nothing going for you. "If you weren't there for me when I was at my worst then you don't deserve me at my best." When I had my years of speech challenges starting with just my incredibly slurred speech, and then the severe stammering and stuttering that made it so hard to get my thoughts out and complete my sentences, who was still interested in what I had to say? And when I was at my lowest and depressed and only able to properly digest 2 foods, who was still there trying to uplift me and give me hope when I needed it? Who had no problem going to the same places to eat with me every time, or was understanding when I had to cancel plans due to not feeling well? When it's just you as raw as possible, see who's still around for you. See who's still cheering for you when you are at your lowest. And the greatest thing happened for me…my best friends emerged as a result.

STOP CONSTANTLY SEEKING APPROVAL
Chapter 48

I see it way too often. People are always looking for the approval of others, especially from those who really don't matter. "A lion doesn't lose sleep over the opinions of sheep." In other words, a lion knows he's a lion, he's the king of the jungle, so what does it matter to him what some sheep think? That's how we all should be living our lives. Especially in today's world of social media, everyone is afraid of posting something that might not get enough likes, or is of an unpopular opinion, or that might not make them look as good as someone else, and I completely understand that fear. I have fallen victim to this at times too. Especially more recently, when it came to me posting my beliefs on health and my beliefs on everything going on in today's world, this drew some backlash. But, I knew what I was speaking to be the truth or at the very least what I believed to be the truth. So, I wasn't going to change who I was or compromise my beliefs to please those who this information offended. My message was going to resonate with whom it was meant to, but it was not up to me to change my beliefs or my actions. Not everyone was ready to hear what I had to say, but the truth must be sought out at all costs. **This is not to say that I have all the answers or that only what I believe is the truth.** But we should all be free to question, as well as speak without fear, in order to arrive at the truth. The same goes for all of my videos of me speaking in general. I was initially worried about being judged for my speech issues. It's easy to fall into the trap of worrying about being judged or fear of failing. I know that all too well. But I know how detrimental this way of thinking is. If we continue with this way of thinking, we end up living a life that isn't ours, but rather one that seeks the approval of everyone else. When you try to please everyone, you end up pleasing no one. So, make sure that you are pleasing the right people, starting with yourself, and others who love you will love you for it. As I say later on, you have to be able to feel the fear and do it anyway. The whole concept of awaiting others' approval is an innate quality; we are born with it, because we are very tribal in nature. And if you aren't part of a tribe or if you aren't approved by others, you are the most "vulnerable" to being attacked by either side, and ultimately you see it as you are going

224

to die first. We overcome this fear by doing what we know is best for us anyway. Don't live the life that others picked out for you, but live YOUR best life. And remember it's better to be hated for who you are than loved for someone you are not.

Be Aware of Blessings Coming Your Way

Whenever I was most in need of a sign or a person to help me keep going, they always seemed to appear, but I had to be ready for it. The world can be a lonely place. There will be times where we feel like it is just us. But having a team can take some of the burden off.

FRIENDS INDIVIDUALLY (MY TEAM)
Chapter 49

When some people say that they don't know where they would be without their friends and family, sometimes they don't truly know what that means. After everything I have been through, I fully understand what that means. As I said, I used to think I could do it all on my own and used to think I didn't need anyone. While independence is a great skill and tool to have, you can't go on forever like that. There's an African proverb that goes, "If you want to go fast, go alone, if you want to go far, go together." Once I was able to find the right people, they enhanced my life so much and made it even more fulfilling! I feel that it's only right to give them the individual shoutouts and recognition that each of them deserve because I really don't know where I'd be without them, and I'm so grateful for them. My hope is that by seeing what qualities are involved in being the best friend, this can help you to build your team.

James and his family:

I have to begin with my best friend in the world James Kass. As you have already read about, I was his counselor for a few years at camp and I knew right away that this kid was special. And although you're not supposed to have favorites, he was my favorite camper. We shared such a special bond right away. He made me realize how the job of a counselor goes beyond just camp. I had such an amazing influence on the campers' lives, and they had a tremendous influence on mine. My bond with James would continue to grow and strengthen into one that can't be broken. He was one of the main motivators when I was in the hospital, without even knowing it. I knew that I couldn't let him down and I had to get back to camp the following summer. His parents requested me so I was able to be his counselor again, and as I spoke about, we had another super fun summer that was essential for me. Thankfully, after that summer, I was able to keep in touch through his mom Jen, who is the sweetest person as well. And soon after in the coming years, we started hanging out more and more until it turned into all the time. The Kass home has become like my second home considering how much time I spend there, and I always feel immediately at ease as soon as I enter.

James never made me feel different or lesser when I was going through my toughest times. He always encouraged me and would tell me how close I am to being better, and he listened to everything I had to say no matter how long it took me to get the words out. At times when I was at my lowest, I knew I couldn't quit because I wanted to show him that if I could overcome this, he could do anything too. He would even do his best to understand my whole holistic health routine and try to understand why I was doing each aspect of the healing process and what I was putting into my body, so this way he could support me with it and take off some of the burden. Even his parents would do their own research to help me get better.

He's always had the key to life and the wisdom beyond his years. Anytime we get together, we discuss our goals and give life to them! He tells me to keep going and to go after all my dreams, and I have inspired him with my mindset. He even copied my home gym idea and often tells me that he wants to get jacked like me and prioritize his health too, since he sees its importance. We have crushed many amazing and fun workouts at my gym Lifetime Fitness, as well as at each of our home gyms! Imitation is the highest form of flattery, and I try to be the best role model and friend possible to him. He's often asking me for advice when it comes to nutrition and working out and shows interest in my deeper holistic health topics and positive life analogies and spirituality. And whenever he asks for advice or when he's going through a rough time, he knows I'm always there for him and he can count on me. As I was saying before, when you are around people who light that spark in you, you can sense it and feel the amazing vibes, and that is how I always knew that James and I would be close. In addition, I have cheered him on at his sports games and he has cheered me on at mine! When I watched him play baseball, I didn't want to put any pressure on him. But as he said I was his good luck charm as he was like a one man show on the field, impressing in both hitting and fielding. And it was the same with me when he watched me play basketball that summer too; I shot lights out as I heard him cheering me on from the sidelines. And even more, when I watched him play football, I was seemingly his good luck charm yet again, and it was as if my presence made him raise his level of play! The craziest thing was during the 2 seasons of going to his varsity football games, every game I went to his team won and every game I missed his team lost—all except for one (which was the last playoff game of his senior season, but in my defense his team had so many injuries, so this was too much for even my good luck presence to overcome lol). Going to every game and watching James play his heart out made me so proud, and it was an absolute blast getting to hang out with Scott and Jen at every game too! (His varsity baseball games also!) We all joked that I wasn't allowed to miss any more games due to my special powers that I seemingly brought James and his team.

Somehow, it's like he can always sense what I need in that moment, whether it be a hug or some positive encouragement or a laugh. Like one time, during the early stages of my healing process after yet another sleepless night due to my stomach feeling horrible, and I was crying all morning from frustration. He had a game that day, and after the game I'm saying bye to his mom; I give her a hug and then I go to give James a high five and he stops me and says, "C'mon, hug!" Knowing just what I needed that day. Or another time when I surprised him at his basketball game and he sees me sitting in the stands and stops shooting around and screams out, "Jared!!" as his eyes light up and he comes running over to me, making me feel so special. Then, there was the time when I had gone three sleepless nights in a row, and he came over that day and encouraged me and made me feel like I had the strength to keep going. Even when it came to writing this book, I would constantly talk to him about it and how it wasn't going to be easy writing about some of the really difficult experiences. He would tell me just what I needed to hear, first being understanding of what I must be feeling and then telling me how he knows I can do it, as I have fought through and conquered every obstacle up to this point. He helped me see my own strength and gave me the confidence to keep going.

James is the most caring, kind individual I know. As I mentioned earlier, a quote I heard recently that totally defines him is, "It's all about who stands in the rain with you when they could be dry if they wanted to." We have the best times whenever we're together, and he lifts my spirits and brings positivity and joy into my life. Whether it's any of the sports we play, filming our awesome YouTube videos, creating our own games, working out together, seeing movies, the amazing karaoke car rides in "Patty," or just chilling and having a deep conversation about life, I can trust him with anything. And I always have his back. We always tell each other that if one of us is upset, then we're both upset. That's what it means to be part of my family. The years when I was going through my speech issues and severe digestive problems, he and his whole family were always there to support me and provide me what I needed! It takes some incredibly special people to really understand me and allow me to feel like part of their family. I know I'm always welcome at the Kass house as Jen has made clear to me, and we have had some incredible dinners and great conversations. When I was going through these really frustrating times during my recovery and couldn't sleep so many nights, I would sometimes become depressed, but as soon as I was in their presence, my whole mood shifted. As I mentioned earlier, I am extremely sensitive when it comes to feeling out energies in the world and know how to listen to what my body is telling me when I am around certain people. The law of attraction demonstrates how when you put out positive energy into the world you will receive similar energies in return. And when you are surrounded by positive energies, you become a more positive person and in a better mood. So, that's how I know I'm in the presence of the right people when I am with their family. They would accommodate me food wise, offer to cook for me, give me emotional support, and would listen to what I was saying without judging me no matter how long it took to get the words out. There would often be a lot of laughs as well. His parents, Jen and Scott, are such warm people. I know I can always count on Jen for heartwarming encouragement to make me feel special and appreciated as well as some profound wisdom, and Scott for his great sense of humor (which cracks me up), amazing insights on every subject, as well as deep conversation. My conversations with Scott and Jen sometimes go all night (even after James has gone to sleep if it's a school night lol). They are amazing listeners and such genuine down to earth people! The great talks with the family on a whole host of topics are something I absolutely look forward to. Being with the family is like medicine for me. James's brother Evan and sister Ryann are such positive and kind people as well, and most of the time they are part of these amazing family dinners too (and I am part of the extended family lol). Evan even appeared in one of our YouTube videos when we had a home run derby. And I can't forget our night run to H Mart to buy some exotic fruit lol. He even decided to use me as one of his job references recently which I was honored to do! Even their cats feel like my own as whenever I sit on the couch I am often welcomed by one of their cats who comes to sit on my lap. I can honestly say I don't know where I would be without James and his family in my life.

The most amazing thing is that when my speech was at its worst, and I could barely even get out a sentence to be understood, this kid who I've known from a young age has always made me believe that I was a superhero to him. He has made me feel like I am special no matter what I sound like and never treated me any differently. One of the most amazing parts about having my best friend be my former camper is that I have been able to serve as a role model for him. As Jen tells me, I have such a positive influence on his life and am like a big brother to him! James and I often say we will always be brothers and despite what blood might say, he is definitely part of my family. And seeing his amazing development is something that I'm proud of because I know that I have played a role in it.

As a result, he inspires me to be the best person I can. One of his best qualities is that whenever I accomplish a personal goal he is almost happier for me than I am for myself, and you can tell how special our friendship is because I am the same way when he accomplishes something. You would think that goal was our own. Like when I touched the rim for the first time he was almost happier for me than I was for myself. And with every food I was able to add back to my diet, and even the tiniest of improvements I would make, were reasons to be ecstatic.

During the summer of 2021 as I hope a lot of the readers know, I decided it was finally time to start our YouTube channel, and who better to do it with me than James? We have such great chemistry off camera and we wanted to spread our positivity and life experience to the world. During his school year and with the school sports, James wasn't able to be in a lot of the videos. But, he still made sure to support the content to the best of his ability and would often tell me how great he thought the job I was doing with the channel and my other social media content was too! We have made some really awesome content and don't plan to stop anytime soon, and have also of course expanded our reach into podcasting. And we're often joined by one of our close and very special friends who I can't forget to mention as well, Ethan Funk, who keeps us laughing non stop. Ethan is incredibly kind and supportive, super fun to be around, and an awesome addition to our team. When it comes to many of our sports competitions or gym vlogs, Ethan is actually often the one behind the ideas for the trio! YouTube/content creation has, and will definitely continue to be, a way that we can continue to enhance our friendship and give us an excuse to do even more fun stuff. Lastly, whenever it's one of my or James's birthdays, this does not get taken lightly as we make sure to make a big deal out of the celebrations!

I love him and his family so much and would do anything for them!

Pictures of me and James over the years...

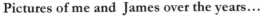

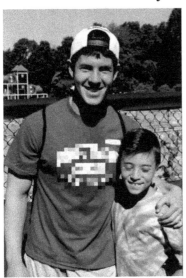
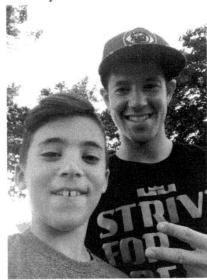

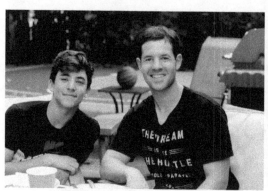

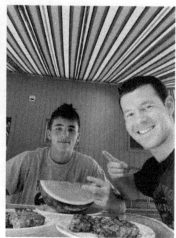

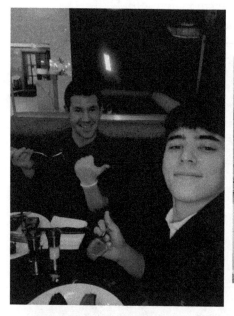

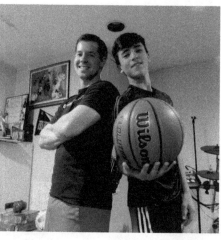

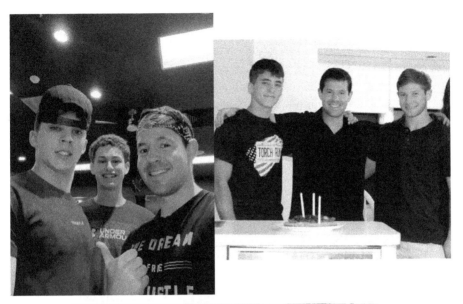

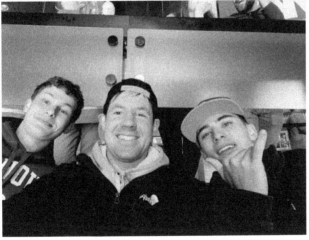

The next few people I don't get to see as often as I did when I initially began writing this book, however, they each played big roles in my healing journey and my life! And I know that if I ever need any of them today, I can always count on them!

Jacob:

Now onto my super close friend and member of my team, Jacob Silverman. We met as well in the summer of 2014 as he was my co counselor. We both had a similar love for working out and also had the passion for working with kids. From making our group sing Nickelback and Aerosmith, and teaching me the line, "That's not what Cornell said" whenever anyone questioned my intelligence or common sense, to making fun of me being like the campers in our group because I act like such a kid, we truly bonded that summer. We had the summer of our lives. Then it was time for our lives to change as we were off to college, but little did I know how much my life was going to change. We called each other a few times before I got sick to see how the other was doing and to reminisce over the great memories that we just made. Then when my illness struck Jacob had no idea, as almost nobody else did, and thought I wasn't responding to his texts because maybe I was just being a jerk. But when he found out that I (the healthiest person he ever knew, the one who wouldn't eat a cookie, and "stupidly" woke up at around 4 am to workout every day lol) got sick, he was in shock. When I came home from the hospital, and a few months later got to see him and hang out, he felt awful, but he kept reminding me that I was a warrior and that if I can make it through that alive I could make it through anything. My speech issues definitely threw him for a loop and at times he didn't know how to respond, but I always knew that he wanted the best for me and his intentions were in the right place, and he just wanted me to get all better as fast as I could. It took some time for me to get my muscles back. But getting back to our workouts with my awesome workout partner definitely helped encourage and motivate me to keep going until I was in the best shape of my life. The summer of 2015 we both went back to camp, and Jacob was truly there for me and by my side. He would help me tell other people what I had been through, since many would have probably felt confused (especially those who knew me before) due to my speech challenges. He would constantly hype me up and tell others about how strong I was and tell me not to worry about what others thought about me, because I know who I am and what I've been through. During the school years when he was at Buffalo and I was at NYU we would text about how much we couldn't wait to be back at camp, and I would update him on my progress with my health as well as my weight room numbers (of course). During the summer of 2017 at camp, we made it our mission to show no fear and to do every competition and special event there was-- whether it was doing the "wrestlemania" and calling ourselves protein man and creatine boy, or dressing up as the Pokemon where he was Ash and I painted my body yellow as Pikachu, and getting my whole group to cheer when he got on stage to do a bottle flip (and landed it). In the summers of 2014 and 2015 we also participated in many of these events such as Simon Sez and dancing contests, and for the counselor makeover

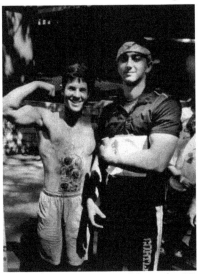 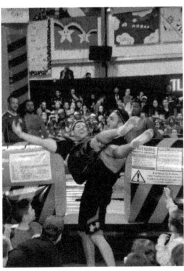

day when I was turned into the Hulk and he was a male cheerleader. Summer of 2017 we also started playing tennis, and the summer of 2020 we picked it up again and made lots of improvement and continued to have intense matches. We even got James and Ethan into it as well, and we all had some fierce tournaments! Jacob and I have had some deep conversations post workout and always have a lot of laughs as well. We even went back to camp one night in 2019 and reminisced outside our old haven. No matter what, we show extreme support for each other's goals. I think I had to convince him at first of the fact that anything was possible. But once I showed him my jump progress and played basketball with him, he was blown away by my skills for someone who is 5'6 and is not your typical looking athlete. Especially after everything I had been through, I had him buying in and believing. He often told me, "You got this" when I was going through my most difficult challenges, as he knew that I was always there for him as well.

And even though we don't see eye to eye on a lot of subjects and we have had some fierce debates, we often find a way to defuse the tension as we know that our friendship is more important than any disagreement we might have. I find this to be a good example that you don't always have to agree with everyone on every topic in order to get along and find the goodness in each other. When you understand the person's intentions and know that they are well meaning, that should be what matters most.

Jake and his family: Next up we have my very good friend Jake Cohen. Jake was also one of my campers, but I first met him in the summer of 2015. Jake didn't know me before my illness yet that didn't matter to him. He treated me like I was his favorite counselor and like I was the coolest guy in the world, an incredible athlete, and most importantly the nicest person. His mom Monica, similar to James's mom, worked at the camp but as a group leader, so this made the friendship seamless. Since that summer I have held so many different roles for Jake, and his family became close to me as well. I was their babysitter for a few years, I became his basketball coach on the team I coached with my uncle, and I also trained him and his brother in basketball for a few years. I gave him the motivation that he needed, including the confidence and encouragement and skills and athleticism that he needed to transform his game. But for me, it's not just about making those who I'm around and those I train better athletes; it's my goal to make them better people who believe in themselves and believe they can achieve anything. And he would reflect that back onto me, telling me he wanted to see me achieve my goals and dunk. Just as I mentioned with James and Jacob, they all wanted me to succeed as much as I wanted to succeed myself. Moreover, he and his family were there for me when I needed them during my illness recovery, always wishing me well and complimenting me on my strength and athletic skills. They didn't care that my speech wasn't what it was "supposed to be," they loved me for who I was as a person. His family brought me into their family as one of their own. And I will never forget it. When I went to his bar mitzvah, it was touching to be given a role in the special occasion. Monica and Brett, Jake's parents have been so supportive of me and have treated me like a rockstar to their family.

Jack and Chase: Lastly, two other important members of my team that I want to give my shoutout to is Jack Pendrick, along with his little brother Chase. I was Jack's counselor in the summer of 2017 and I started babysitting for him and his brother as well, and our friendship has grown each year. They accepted me for who I was and always put a smile on my face whenever I needed them. I've been to their birthday parties and acted as one of the kids as they said. And when I was Jack's counselor we had so many great times and amazing laughs, including our competitiveness in sports at camp and having deep conversations about life and everything that I had been through. Years later, when I was trying to heal my body, they were always encouraging me by telling me how strong I was. They were some of my biggest fans, cheering me on in my athletic and fitness journey, telling all their friends about me and hoping that I would get better. Whenever I babysat for them, we always had a blast as they knew they could count on me to take the stress away from whatever they were going through and help them have the best time. From soccer tournaments, FIFA and 2K, flag football, keep away, laser tag, and making them special drinks and food, we definitely knew how to create tons of fun!

As you can see, this forms my team along with my brothers and parents and the rest of my family. I have spoken about how my relationships with my parents, siblings, grandparents, aunts, uncles, and friends were vital to my development and healing; they have always been there for me, and I feel this is a good place to also show my appreciation for my cousins who have always played a huge role in my life as well: Adam for always putting the funniest spin on things and our talks about sports; Amanda always being so sweet and positive and taking the time to listen to what I have to say; and Dylan always keeping me laughing, talking sports, going to the movies and working out together!

LIFETIME FITNESS CREW

Although I wouldn't be able to single any one person out, my circle of important connections that I've made wouldn't feel complete without mentioning my gym crew at Lifetime Fitness. If you've watched any of my gym vlogs, or heard various of my podcasts, chances are you've already met some of these awesome people. My gym squad has been pivotal in my healing journey because by having these people whom I talk to on a daily basis and who support my journeys—whether on social media, healing journey or dunk/athletic journey—and having a community to motivate each other—is amazing and satisfies my need for like minded connections, similar to how working at camp did! Moreover, it's pretty unbelievable to see how while going through all of my speech challenges, I've been able to meet and connect with so many people on a deep level every single day. I even often get referred to as the "mayor of Lifetime" because of how many people know me there lol (as James once said every person between ages 15 and 60 knows me there)! Sometimes it even takes me an extra hour just to get through my workout because I get involved in so many conversations with all different kinds of people. I've discovered that when people have this common ground of the gym, it sometimes leads to the most unlikely connections being formed. And although as I mentioned I prefer to keep a super small inner circle, I've found that having a nice outer circle of connections can be super important as well! We also have a pretty consistent daily sauna crew full of awesome conversations. As Chance Garton spoke about on my podcast, doing all this speaking as a form of communication has been important for me in clearing out my throat chakra energy, so in other words, everything that I've been doing and all of these friendships and connections have actually been feeding into my healing journey as well! Also this constant feedback I was receiving every day fueled my desire to be better with everything I was doing. As I mentioned earlier, for a period of time I was thinking that I had to be fully healed in order for everything I was saying and doing to matter—but what I began to learn through all of my special connections was that I was already impacting plenty of people, and people valued what I was saying and valued me as a person, regardless of what I was going through and what I sounded like!

FEELING LIKE A BURDEN AT TIMES...
Chapter 50

There were a lot of times when I was going through my healing process when I thought of myself as a burden. This is part of the irrational thinking that we formulate sometimes. There were days when I would get so frustrated or depressed, but instead of reaching out to friends or family to talk to, I wouldn't want to bother them with my problems. After all, I was always the one who was supposed to be happy and optimistic. There's a scene from the movie, *Robots* when the main character Rodney says, "If you burden your friends, soon you won't have any." Then the character voiced by late comedian Robin Williams says, "What are you a fortune cookie? That's what friends are for." That's the truth, and I realized that whenever I would speak to a friend or a family member about what I was going through, I almost always felt better afterwards, almost as if they were taking on some of my stress and sharing it, in turn making it a lighter load for me to carry. It's not easy to reach out for help when we are in need, but it is the best thing for you to do. And most of the time if you have the right inner circle, they will be so thankful that you did reach out because they care about you and know you would do the same for them.

HOW I FEEL WHEN IT COMES TO MY SPEECH
Chapter 51

I dealt with a lot of emotional stuff when it came to my speech issues. I would sometimes stammer and stutter to the point where I didn't even get to say what I wanted. It wasn't that I couldn't think of what I wanted to say, but I just couldn't get it out due to what was going on with my brain. Or, when my slurred speech was at its worst I would need to repeat myself constantly and slow it all down. This was so frustrating to have to go through day after day for years. Sometimes I would start crying and other times the sadness and frustration would just boil up inside of me, as I was trying to show those around me that I was stronger than what I was going through. I can handle anything. But crying is not a sign of weakness, it shows that you've been staying strong for too long and is a necessary release at times. I would tell myself to be thankful that I'm still breathing and that's what mattered most, as well as to trust God's plans. I'm still alive for a reason, and I have to be grateful for all that I do have rather than focus on what I don't. Most people take these normal human functions for granted; that's not to say that they don't appreciate the life they've been given, but you just don't think you could ever lose them. I wasn't able to talk properly, couldn't digest foods properly, didn't have the optimal energy levels, I was seeing things as "tilted," yet every day I made an effort to be grateful. I was more thankful than ever for my best friends and for my family, who always made sure to make me feel like no matter what I was going through I was still a great person. I tried to tell myself that God was just testing me and that I wouldn't have been given these challenges if I couldn't overcome them. Maybe I had to use this to show others what humans are truly capable of. Even when it seems like nothing is going right, you can still accomplish great things and you can still be the best person.

Sometimes I was ridiculed for my speech problems early on by little kids who didn't know better, as well as some people who I thought were my friends at the time. They turned out to be people who weren't really there for me and I had to get them out of my life. But, I also couldn't totally avoid these situations, so I had to remind myself that they didn't know my story and that I would get all better—it was just going to take some time.

There were so many times when I would get so frustrated and either want to stop talking or pull out my phone and just type what I was trying to say, but I knew I couldn't let the people around me down. I had to show them and myself that I was mentally tough enough to endure the stress even if I was crying inside and behind closed doors. But this made me infinitely grateful for those who didn't care what I sounded like and just wanted to be with me.

Some people would bring up my speech issues in conversation without me bringing it up, which made me very insecure and uncomfortable. Of course it was always nice when someone would give me a genuine compliment or give me their full support and tell me or show me that they truly didn't mind my speech issues, as they wanted to hear what I had to say. Those things of course I always welcomed. But, when you start talking about how much I stammer and stutter and how well you can or can't understand me, that's gonna make me think more about it and mess with my head. Sometimes people would tell me I should see a different medical doctor even after I told them that they would only make things worse—as I had experienced—by recommending anti-anxiety medication or just charging me money to give me "treatment" that wouldn't work. I wasn't looking for anyone else to "fix me" or tell me how "my body was messed up." I knew what I was doing by embracing natural medicine and getting to the root of my issues. This was monumental and was going to take a seriously long time to heal. I just needed support. I didn't need suggestions on what I should be doing because if I wanted those I would have asked.

Moreover, the more I started putting out content on social media, being someone who has speech difficulties and speaking these "controversial hard truths" left me open to plenty of criticism from nasty comments, from people who didn't know my whole story and how hard it was to even put myself out there every day for people to hear. For all of the incredibly kind comments I would get, I also received some hurtful comments with regards to my speech. As Amanda Porta said when she came on my podcast, "Your light is going to irritate others' demons." I wasn't going to let these comments stop me from following my purpose and from realizing how special I am. But, the amazing thing about starting the podcast and making all these YouTube videos while being on my healing journey—it was extremely therapeutic and I actually started to love the way I sounded even with all my "flaws." I began to have empathy for myself and I loved myself and became super proud of myself knowing how difficult this was to do. Many people who don't have speech issues are afraid to speak on camera, but here I was doing it all the time. And the more guests I started to have on and the more people who I'd connect with at my gym, the more I realized how many people were cool with it and wanted to hear me no matter how I sounded. I would build more strength and courage each time I overcame this challenge and had a long conversation. And when the comments from others who dealt with their own speech issues telling me how inspiring what I was doing started to come in, this helped me realize that even though these seeming "flaws" and definite challenges were tough, and it wasn't always easy to see the positive side of them, maybe I was actually the perfect person to be dealing with them. And when you combine that with the understanding that the body is always perfect in its responses, there must have been a reason I was dealing with these speech "issues," so in its own weird kind of way it was actually perfect for me. This doesn't mean that it was any less difficult and that my life wouldn't be "easier" without them, but maybe this was all part of my spiritual path! And as Chance Garton said when he came on my podcast, I was "making the obstacle the way!" And for the people who couldn't deal with them, those probably weren't my type of people anyway. I eventually reached this special place where I loved myself with all my flaws, (although this doesn't mean I wasn't doing everything I could to make them better); this was an important step in my growth as a person and my healing journey. When you truly love yourself, and can have acceptance of yourself and the things that can't be changed, the opinions of others stop mattering as much!

Thankfully, some people always managed to make me feel better. People like my brother Brandon, and James always knew how to brighten my outlook and give me the perspective and positivity that I needed. They wouldn't make me feel different for my speech issues and would only give encouragement when I would feel bad about how hard it was for me to be understood. When it came to Brandon, he and I used to talk non stop for hours back before any of this happened so it must have been difficult for him to adjust to this, but he didn't flinch. And James, who I had met the summer before all this happened, did not change one bit towards me either—I was still the same to him. Both allowed me the time I needed to get out what I had to say.

There is truly something to be said for the people who were in my life when everything was going wrong with my health. A true friend is someone who you know you can be comfortable around no matter what is going on in your life, and you know that they'll support you. I tear up sometimes just thinking about my best friends and family because what they mean to me can't be put into words, and I am just so blessed to have such wonderful people in my life.

MY 6TH SENSE
Chapter 52

Ever since going through all of my health struggles, I feel like this has made me a much more empathetic person. I can really feel and understand the challenges that people go through. They say that when one ability is taken away, others become enhanced. I have had seemingly every ability taken away from me in these past few years at one point or another, and I really feel that I've had a changed perspective and appreciation for life as a result.

Three examples of this are as follows: First, while going through my speech difficulties, whether from the slurred speech or the stammering and stuttering at times making me afraid to speak at all, I became a better listener. I have always been known to be a good listener, always enjoying helping others get through their toughest of problems because I'm never one to distract myself when friends are speaking. But not being able to say what I want all the time has forced me to listen to the emotion that one speaks with and sense what is truly going on in their lives. It also enhanced my writing ability as I needed another form and outlet of expressing myself.

Next, not being able to eat basically any food for quite some time forced me to become an expert at listening to my body. I am so in tune with how foods feel to me now. And I have also become an expert in digestion because of all the tireless research I've done to get myself feeling better. I am aware of how every action I take makes me feel. And I am constantly asking myself whether what I am doing is contributing to my overall positive health—body, spirit, and mind, or whether it is contributing to toxicity. These revelations would not have occurred had I not had these abilities taken away.

Moreover, having gone through all of these issues led to a surge in anxiety and depression, which at times felt like I couldn't handle what life was throwing at me. I would just cry or be so wound up in my thoughts while realizing how disheartening everything was. I have often dealt with anxiety throughout my life and am one who is constantly overthinking things and wanting everything to be perfect, which also probably explains my work ethic. If you want everything to be perfect you will do whatever it takes, which sometimes leads you to going overboard. I now understand that my anxiety just means that I care so much and care extra about certain things. If I am anxious before a game, it just means I really want to play well because I care about that game. If I am anxious about making sure that my plans follow through when seeing a friend, it just means that I really care about that friend and really want the plans to go well. If I'm anxious about dying (even though I believe we are all eternal spiritual beings and don't believe that death is "the end") or getting "sick" again, that means I love living and am grateful for my health. One way to look at anxiety is to see it as your mind is driving you crazy, but on the other hand, it is making sure that you are remembering how much that thing means to you. Every feeling and emotion has a reason for being there. When you are able to change perspective like that, it helps you deal with challenges so much better and releases some of the fear.

Having gone through all of the struggles that I have at such a young age has made me a much deeper person and has taught me life lessons that most will never learn. It has added layers to me. I am able to be more passionate about what I do, and I can love and appreciate others who have made my life better and one worth living.

SAY YES TO LIFE
Chapter 53

When I first started having my severe speech challenges, which was something that I had never dealt with nor did I ever think I would have to deal with, it made me afraid to see people…even friends who I knew would love to see me no matter what was wrong. At times I really just wanted to be alone. But this is no way to live. You have to understand that you matter, you are inspiring others by continuing to move forward. And I don't care if you have millions of fans and followers or just one friend; if you are relevant to someone, then you are relevant, and your actions will speak louder than your words. In my case this was literally how I had to approach my life. I was never really a vocal leader (interestingly enough, one of my issues while playing point guard in high school was that my coaches and teammates always told me I wasn't loud enough especially when calling the plays), but I did always love to talk to people that I felt close with. Many times and days when I didn't feel up to going outside or seeing people, I would decide to stop feeling bad for myself and make what I knew was the right decision. Yes, it was frustrating and yes it was difficult, but I showed myself and others around me that I would not be defined by what I couldn't do and instead would accomplish what needed to be done.

By going outside of my comfort zone, I was exposing myself to being made fun of by people who didn't know my story or to difficulties with frightening circumstances even as simple as ordering food and not being understood. But I was going to say yes to life again. By opening myself up, I was also opening myself up to some of the kindest actions taken by my friends and family. They wanted me to know that they were not going to treat me any differently, and they reminded me how much I matter, and that they still need me to be the fun, loving and encouraging person in their lives that they were used to. And by putting myself out there and showing my story online through my posts and videos, I ended up making numerous connections (many of these connections came from the sauna and at my gym as I stated before) which led me to inspiring so many people! I did a podcast with Jake Moscato (and his co-host Zach

Cummings) whom I became friendly with at my gym, and one with Victor, my naturopath, and as many of you know by now, this then led to my own podcast taking off as part of my YouTube channel. As many guests would say to me, they didn't know any other podcasters who would put their speech challenges on display and be completely unphased. They said how much courage it takes even for the "normal person" to put out a podcast. So, I basically started revolving much of my life around speaking…while having tremendous "speech issues." I ended up connecting with a lot of people and have been told by many that my story is the most inspiring one they have ever heard. So just by putting myself out there and stepping out of my comfort zone, I was showing people what it takes to overcome anything!

There were times when I didn't feel up to going to the gym whether from digestion issues or lack of energy, or having just gotten over a sleepless night. Sometimes I did need to listen to my body and give in to the rest. But, if it wasn't that bad and I could push through it, I would tell myself on the way there that I was going to "suffer beautifully" and that if I could win this part of my day, then something would be accomplished. This is also why it is so important to remember the little wins and tiny things to be appreciative for. Maybe the full day wasn't a great one, maybe someone said something nasty to you, or maybe you weren't feeling your best, but if you can recall the positives such as you had a great workout or someone smiled at you or that you have a roof over your head and breath in your body, then you are winning. A lot of small daily wins will eventually add up. Don't let your circumstances define what you do. Let your character and actions define who you are, and you dictate what you will be doing.

Going along these same lines, looking back at the end of 2021 and into 2022, one of my former campers and now one of my friends, Zak Labib, asked me if I wanted to coach his basketball team. In past years I had always coached with my Uncle David as I coached my cousin Dylan. We would have a great time and made it to the championship twice with me as the assistant coach. However, this year Dylan wasn't playing. Aside from head coaching sports league at camp from 2014-2017 (and doing an amazing job if I do say so myself lol), I hadn't been a head coach and wasn't eager to, especially since now having the more difficult speech challenges with the stammer and stutter. But, the opportunity was presented to me so I decided to take on the challenge. The first 2 games I stayed mostly reserved in an effort to not say a lot so that the kids wouldn't notice my speech issues. One of the other kids on the team who I developed a close bond with, Isaac, told me how the team needed me to speak more and how he knew how much I could help them. He promised me that everyone decided that I was the best leader and the team needed me, and they all wanted to hear what I had to say. So, I decided I was up for the challenge and even started making pregame speeches before games. I made an effort to talk to the kids as much as I could and they absolutely loved having me as a coach. This was an example of making my life part of my medicine!

OPPOSITE OF ADULTS...
Chapter 54

Kids are amazing. There is so much to be learned from them. For starters, they are masters of living in the moment. One minute they could be upset and crying and the next running around with joy and laughter, completely forgetting about what made them upset. They also know how to have fun as they are naturally creative. They can make up a great game in a short amount of time and no matter how simple it sounds, they can have the most fun playing it. Kids will celebrate every little great thing that happens. Something as simple as chicken nuggets for lunch is enough to get kids high fiving and jumping up and down. Kids will dream the biggest dreams and not care what others tell them "can't" be done, because they value the imagination. They don't care what seems realistic or not, because they believe they can accomplish anything. Every year since I was a camp counselor I have always prided myself on being a kid and used to be considered as another "camper" in my group. I wanted to be a role model for these kids and to inspire them. They always told me that I was the best because "I get them" and I understood them. Whenever there was a problem, I would have this unbelievable ability to put myself in their shoes and treat them the way I would have wanted to be treated. In other words, I tried to become the hero that I needed (and loved) when I was younger.

And in recent years this has held up, as I have had numerous former campers of mine (referring to ones who I hadn't been totally in touch with) who would reach out to me when they were going through some depression. They came to me because they felt I was the only one who could help them through it. And after these talks they would tell me how much better they felt. I am 1000% a kid at heart, and I feel like and try to stay a kid because of all the reasons I mentioned. Of course I typically act more mature and know how to be more serious and turn the switch, but I try to take the best qualities from kids and employ them with my own behavior. I never really felt like an adult because I never wanted to get away from the things I love, never wanted to abandon my creativity and imagination and appreciation for all the little things in life.

Fight Through It

Whenever I find myself taking things too seriously, I know I have to get back to the little Jared who just did things because they were fun. I love creating games when I'm with my friends, and I never stopped believing that anything is possible. I never curse because I don't like the way those words make ME feel (not saying you have to be the same way). I enjoy good clean fun and try to be an optimist as best as possible. Life will occasionally try to bring you down and tell you not to be happy. And society will try to get you to "grow up" and tell you to sit down and shut up and listen to what we say, and will tell you to take a job you do not like and to go out drinking and do drugs for fun because "you want to escape from life." Of course life has responsibilities and no one can be happy all the time. But, I'm telling you to act younger and be a kid again. Life has so many great moments as long as you are open to them. It's meant to be lived to the fullest, and you are supposed to enjoy yourself and have fun with what you are doing. It's okay to get knocked down, but it's not okay to stay down. The person who never gets knocked down will never know what it's like to have to pick themselves up again and to claw their way back up. Be like the kid who gets back up on the bike every time after falling and scraping his knee, but doesn't let it deter him. Be like the kid who keeps shooting that basketball even though he just missed his last 100 shots, but believes that the next shot is going in. I appreciate the bountiful positivity that acting like a "kid" gives me, and I think everyone could benefit from these qualities no matter what age you are.

2018 SUMMER DOWNFALL
Chapter 55

Sometimes You Just Have to Let Go

Going into the summer of 2018, my health struggles were hitting their peak. Every food I ate was still causing me severe issues, my stammering and stuttering speech issues were at their worst, and my balance issues had started as well. The worst part was we had zero clue as to what was going on. The year was filled with going to so many doctors and figuring out nothing, while still trying to get through school and hopefully be able to make it back to camp for the summer. Each doctor would have their own theory that led us nowhere. Meanwhile I wanted to be a preteen travel program counselor this summer for the first time, which meant I would be going on overnight trips with kids who I had from the previous two summers. Although most of my campers whom I knew so well and had become so close with were no longer there, I was excited to have the opportunity to do what I had done as a camper, but to have the experience from the counselor's perspective. Camp was always my happy place; when everything during the year seemed to be going awry, I always had the summer camp to look forward to. After much planning how I was going to do a travel program in spite of all my health issues getting worse, we figured it out. My mom was going to cook my food basically every day, and when it came to the overnights I would store my food in a YETI. Just as I always had done, I was going to make the best of everything. I wouldn't let my circumstances dictate the outcome, and I was going to have a fun summer. Back when I was a preteen camper myself during my first year, I would sometimes get really homesick and cry, but I slowly overcame my fear of being away from home. Although this time, I really hadn't spent a night away from home since my few weeks stint at Cornell. So I wanted to prove to myself that I could do it. Another goal was to make any campers who might feel the same way that I did comfortable in knowing that they could talk to me if they were nervous at all, and that I would be there for them, and that it's okay to be nervous. That's what it's all about, being the guy who you needed when you were younger. Going into the summer, I was told by so many parents how their kids were absolutely thrilled that I was going to be their counselor and how amazing this made the parents feel as well that I was their kids' counselor. I guess I had really developed quite a great reputation at the camp.

The first few weeks of camp went pretty well. We went on some fun trips and I was doing the best I could to manage my symptoms, and the days spent at camp were fun too. Then came the first overnight trip to New Jersey and Six Flags. I made it through with flying colors, proving to myself that I could do it. I even went to the hotel gym early on day 2 at 5:00 am for my usual workout (at that time I was still waking up super early every day). I couldn't miss that just because I was away with camp. The other counselors were all very supportive of everything I was going through and I really appreciated that.

A few days after that overnight trip, yet another difficult challenge was presented to me and yet another situation that was out of my control. A misunderstanding occurred which quickly got blown out of proportion. And this led to a disagreement with the upper staff. Ultimately I felt like I wasn't respected and that my voice wasn't being heard. After 17 years at this camp, I felt like this was the one time my character was attacked, and they should have known who I was and what I was all about. After all I had done for the camp and all they had done for me, things were not the same anymore. My campers were deeply hurt and I felt betrayed by the place I loved.

After the end of that summer, I realized that I really didn't deserve that disrespect. This was always my favorite place on earth, but I felt abandoned by it. I deserved to be around people who loved me and treated me the way I deserved to be treated. I always thought I would be at that camp my whole life. It held and still holds such a special place in my heart. It was one of the hardest decisions of my life, but for a lot of reasons I felt it didn't make sense for me to go back the following summer. In addition, most of my favorite people and now my best friends were no longer there, and if I did go back I would be trying to replicate the amazing summers of the past which I didn't think would be possible. I was trying hard to hold onto the place that I loved, but it wasn't serving its purpose anymore. I still love and will always love that camp and all the amazing things it has done for me. And the impact that I had on that place goes so deep. Thankfully, I feel that I was able to take the best people who now are my best friends from camp and create camp-like fun on our own. All of the incredible memories will never die as I can take them with me, and I will always cherish them.

As I said earlier, I think that everything happens for a reason, yet we often don't see that reason in the moment. Although it was tough (and I still miss those times), I knew I had to move on. It would've been much more difficult to ever leave if that hadn't happened, but truthfully maybe it was time to work on creating new experiences outside of my comfort zone and work on growing my friendships on my own. I learned the lesson that it's important not to hang onto something just because it held value in the past. Sometimes, you have to take the best aspects from that place, thank them for what they've given you in the past, take the amazing memories with you and use them to create amazing experiences on your own. I would've been stuck trying to create memories and trying to replicate past summers without the people I loved. I would've felt trapped working for people who didn't value my contributions anymore and didn't respect my dedication to the campers. The camp was just a place; it didn't mean that I couldn't have fun without it or that I couldn't use what I learned there to impact the lives of children and other people outside of it. The same thing goes for people who no longer make you happy. You can't hang onto them just because they used to be nice to you in the past. You have to let go and do what's best for you now. Sometimes you need an event to show you the door out as a way to open up new doors to other adventures.

The summers since really turned out amazingly fun as I was growing my friendships and truly working on myself. Of course there was still the healing process and challenging times I was going through, but I had the ability to take the amazing people from the camp, learn from the fun I had there and transform it into the most fun I ever had with my friends. It was truly incredible. Whether it was my idea of color war at my house with me and James versus Jacob and Jake and making a full night of it in

2019, or making tons of awesome YouTube content with James and Ethan Funk, football and track workouts with James, having super fun birthday celebrations, a number of awesome lunches and dinners, riding bikes, playing basketball and just goofing around living in the moment—or playing basketball and hanging out with Brandon and spending more time with family while doing my own training and healing and working towards my career goals—I definitely figured out how to bring the camp fun to my life! The fun trio of me, James, and Ethan even started taking camp-like trips to places like Splish Splash, bowling, and Top Golf!

THE START OF A NEW ERA: JARED AND JAMES CHANNEL

Chapter 56

At the end of 2019, I made the decision to start writing this book and worked on it diligently over the next few years. And, in the summer of 2021 James and I decided it was time to start our YouTube channel! This way I could spread my impact on all of the topics I'm passionate about and hope for it to go worldwide. And I started becoming consistent with posting to all of my social media platforms-Instagram Facebook Snapchat and TikTok. This would not have been possible had I not left the camp. Not surprisingly, many of my early followers and biggest supporters just happened to be my former campers. This shows how deep my impact went. I had no prior filmmaking experience and had never really used a camera before. I had never studied this stuff in college. Yet I taught myself how to do it all, and within a few months I was making some incredible content (if I do say so myself). I have never done anything without putting forth my best effort, and this was no different. The original plan was actually to wait until I was feeling all better to start the channel and start posting more on social media. But, I then realized how many people I could be helping and impacting right now. I said to James I don't care if people make fun of me, if this helps one person then it's worth it to me. I said how even if we only get a few followers and views, if we can make an impact on just one person, it would be worth it. At the very least it would be a lot of fun, and at most it could be life changing for us and whoever joins us for the ride. I made the decision to get over my fears of speaking to the camera and to open myself up to being judged by all these people. And even when James has been too busy with school and sports (he still supports the channel but is unable to be in many of the videos), I have been continuing to make full length videos/podcasts every week (YouTube/Spotify/Rumble/Apple Podcast etc.), plenty of short clips to every platform multiple times every day, all by myself most of the time with no help, even while continuing my healing process. I use these platforms as a tool to spread my impact on a wider scale and as a form of self-expression and creativity. As El Stone aka The Ancient Ninja spoke about when she came on my podcast, "the matrix" is ultimately within each of us—so it's up to us to alchemize everything and every situation however suits us best. That's why I don't see social media or all this technology as all bad or all good; it all depends on the person using it and what they are using it for. (I don't love all aspects of these platforms themselves, but they are tools with potential for good when used the right way). I wanted to show people and myself that I could do it. And these efforts are paying off as the channel continues to grow. I love speaking on a variety of topics in the hopes of helping people through their challenges, while ultimately spreading messages of love and positivity, helping people vibrate at higher frequencies, entertaining and inspiring through sports/weight training and vlogs, as well as empowering and encouraging people to believe in themselves more. I also like to stir the pot when it comes to speaking some hard truths that I believe are important to get out there, even if it ruffles some feathers. What I love about being a content creator (and why I hope to do this full time) is that I have full creative control; if I want to make a video of me working out or playing basketball I can do that, and the very next video can be a hard truth topic; I am not limited at all! In case you haven't realized by now, I have various interests and am passionate about a bunch of different things, so rather than limit myself to one job for my whole life as is the "conventional way," I can do them all at the same time. I know I can always rely on myself so I don't need some boss or coach whom I disagree with telling me what I can and can't do! Plus, there are various avenues to branch off into if I ever choose to as well. And as I constantly remind myself and my followers, my top priority is not about how many views or likes a post gets; those things are cool but are more of a bonus and an awesome reward. Of course I do hope to attain those things, but I want to get there the right way instead of the fast way! The most important thing is making an impact on people's lives, being my genuine authentic self, and being proud of the content I produce (as well as having fun with it). And the more lives I impact and help positively change, the more those bonuses will come!

Rabbit Hole Roundup

Going along these lines of content creation, I can't forget to mention the amazing work that RJ aka TheNoodnick, a new good friend of mine, and I have done with our Rabbit Hole Roundup podcast (I originally wanted to keep it all on the Jared and James channel, but I recently created separate accounts for my "truther"/hard truths content on certain platforms due to the shadowbanning and censorship. As Sam Tripoli says, "You don't change the game...you have to beat the game," so I believe this new setup gives me the best chance at success, even though it's not what I prefer.) A few months prior to the release of this book, I was approached by RJ at the gym (he's a calisthenics master) who recognized me from appearing on another podcast which he had gone on as well. We got into talking and an instant connection was made. We bonded over our love of conspiracy and truth seeking topics, in addition to fitness. And after I had him on my podcast once, I got a call a few days later from RJ telling me that his inner voice was telling him that he and I were meant to start up a weekly podcast. I'm a picky guy as I spoke about when it comes to whom I truly let into my life and become part of my circle, especially with someone who I'm going to be working with and seeing often...but I had a good feeling about this. Thus, the Rabbit Hole Roundup was created, and just a few months in and we are absolutely crushing it and having so much fun with it as well. I expect many more good things to emerge from this, and I believe that our strong bond will continue to grow as well! And it's always an added bonus when RJ's girlfriend Kim joins us for some awesome conversations too, as well as an occasional gym workout together. RJ is one of the nicest, most supportive, down to Earth people I know, and it's an honor to be working with him on putting out this amazing content! Update: Although he had too much going on to stick with it full time, he helped me start a really cool type of conversation/concept on the channel, so even when I go solo or have guests on, the spirit of the Rabbit Hole Roundup does not get lost! And we still have plenty of awesome conversations and workouts at the gym, and he's hoping to be back when he has more time or at the very least join me for special episodes!

SLOW AND SMALL PROGRESS IS STILL PROGRESS

Chapter 57

To get to where you want, you have to be willing to put in the time. How much time? However long it takes. We cannot give up at the first feelings of doubts or when we experience setbacks, or when it gets hard. Other people will try to convince you that what you are doing is impossible, and this just means that they are not willing to put up with the rejections and trials and tribulations that come along during the journey. Remember that there is no glory in being a victim. Become a victor and do your best to overcome your circumstances. There will always be excuses available and some are even valid, but that doesn't mean you have to use them. As Rocky Balboa said, "Nobody is gonna hit as hard as life, but it ain't about how hard you can hit. It's about how hard you can get hit and keep moving forward. How much you can take and keep moving forward. That's how winning is done." If you are doing something tiny to improve every single day, eventually those consistent efforts built up over a long period of time will lead to huge gains. The stonecutter's credo reads "When nothing seems to help, I go look at the stonecutter hammering away at his rock, perhaps a hundred times without as much as a crack showing in it. Yet at the hundred and first blow it will split in two and I know it was not that blow that did it, but all that had gone before." When times get tough, look back at how far you've come and remember that your 101st blow could be just around the corner.

LIFE IS NOT OBLIGATED TO BE "FAIR," BUT IF YOU ARE OPEN TO LEARNING IT WILL BE THE BEST TEACHER

Chapter 58

One of my favorite pressure releasing mottos is "I either win or I learn." In other words there is no losing, there is no wasted time, there are no bad games or bad experiences, because in every loss or every negative experience there is always something to be learned. As I mentioned earlier, from 8th grade onward, one of my main passions was health and wellness in order to become the best athlete and best person I could possibly be. I have never even had a piece of "junk food" or food that I consider to be unhealthy since the 8th grade. My body is my temple and I don't want to do anything that can damage it.

Moreover, I always wanted to be a role model, so to me if I was trying to show kids and adults as well who look up to me the importance of a healthy lifestyle, it would be hypocritical to be doing things like getting drunk and eating garbage. I never curse (unless I'm quoting someone or am super angry lol). I am someone who tries to live my life by principles. This helps guide my decision making in difficult times as I'm always trying to be the best version of myself.

So, as you can tell, I thought I was doing everything in my power to stay healthy, not get sick, and bulletproof my body. Although I now realize that there are SO MANY more aspects of health such as detoxification, getting sleep, and taking into account the importance of relationships with people, meditation and spiritual health, etc. Even in spite of not knowing these things, I was still doing my best to take control over my health and clearly I was doing much more than the average teenager. So it came as such a shock when I was the one who got so sick. It didn't seem fair and it didn't make sense. How could this happen to me? I was supposed to be the healthy one. Over the years, I saw all my peers eating whatever they wanted and participating in many harmful behaviors. Was I doing something wrong? As I mentioned earlier, in hindsight there are many potential causes of why I got so sick in the first place. As much as I tried to control things, I couldn't control the sequence of events that spiraled out of control. I couldn't control the toxins that had accumulated in my body that I had yet to learn about. I never even thought about a toxic input. Going along those lines, there's a really interesting concept that Alec Zeck once mentioned in a podcast which is that, when you don't know about something, it can't be your responsibility. So, if you find $5000 in your backyard; prior to knowing this money was there, it wasn't your responsibility. Same thing goes for your life decisions.

But, no matter how hard you try, things don't always happen the way they're "supposed to" or the way YOU think they are supposed to, because I now believe the universe is always working in your favor as long as you're continuing to strive towards your best self. But this was one of the hardest lessons I had to learn. I couldn't control everything…as much as I tried. **The hardest worker doesn't always get the spot on the team, and bad things happen to good people**. However, accepting this does not mean that you should not be doing everything in your power to control what you can. You do have a lot of control over your life and your health and the direction that your life takes, but after you have put the work in and done what you are supposed to do, some things are out of your control. Just because you can't achieve perfection does not mean you should stop trying, or just because something bad happened to you does not mean you should stop being a good person or stop giving your best effort. It's up to us to make meaning out of our struggles and to find the reason. "I either win or I learn."

EVERYTHING HAPPENS FOR A REASON

Chapter 59

"Things turn out best for the people who make the best of the way things work out"-John Wooden

You can either sit around wondering why something bad happened to you and complain about it, or you can search for the meaning and reason behind it! And if all else fails, you go out and make meaning out of it. IT IS NOT EASY. But once you have accepted what has happened to you and accepted the challenge of getting through it, then you can begin to discover the purpose in the challenge. This mindset can help you get through almost anything that the world hands you.

As I have gotten in touch with my inner spirituality throughout my healing journey, I have come to the conclusion that we are all vessels of God. We are all connected and have God consciousness within us. However, we also have what's called free will. So, I believe the universe and God are always going to give you the opportunities to reach your highest self, but then it's up to your own choices through free will to make the right decisions. The thing is, even if you don't believe the universe is out there doing things for you or you don't believe that things "really" do happen for a reason, acting as if they do will still benefit you. It is still in your best interests because when you act like things are happening the way they are supposed to, you turn your attitude towards "bad" situations around and start seeing the good in the midst of chaos. For instance, let's look at a sequence of events for me. In 2014 I had the best time at camp that summer and met my future best friend James. Now, looking back I see that God made this connection happen for when I would need a best friend most. And I believe that many connections and friendships I've made have all seemed to happen at just the time I needed them to. And at first cultivating these friendships wasn't easy, but I worked at it and made it happen, and now I have the best friends in the world and exactly what I needed to get me through some of the most difficult times. I had other friends during this time who weren't right for me. They weren't able to live up to the high standards that I hold for those whom I allow into my life and my inner circle. Maybe this was the universe's way of demonstrating to me how much I leveled up and outgrew those people. Going through the toughest of times showed me who my family was and which friends were to become my family. Sometimes that's what it takes.

Looking at my college situation from a different lens…because I didn't finish up at Cornell, I came home and had the opportunity to live my college life at home. This gave me the time I wanted to spend with my family and brothers, and allowed me to cultivate the relationships with my friends which might not have happened had I been away. This also gave me a chance to work on myself more than ever. I was able to go to my favorite gym all the time and work on my vertical jump and all of my sports skills. I became a better athlete than ever, even though I had to come back from the basement. Maybe, I would have gotten lonely at Cornell and wouldn't have discovered the things I'm truly passionate about. And maybe I would never have improved at these passions. Maybe I would have gotten so stressed out but stuck with studying things I didn't want to (and probably would've become jaded by all the indoctrination once I woke up to the "matrix" that we're all living in lol). Maybe I wouldn't have realized how much I love influencing and inspiring others. Maybe everything I went through with my health was there to give me the platform I needed to help others through whatever they are experiencing, as well as give me the compassion and empathy I needed to be the best friend and person I could be. Now I can motivate and inspire more people than ever to truly believe that anything is possible. First I had to prove it to myself, and now I'm telling the world. Maybe the trauma I went through was showing me that you don't need circumstances to be perfect to still accomplish big things and that nothing worth having comes easy. Yes, my life veered far off from the "plan." I had to put things off in order to reclaim my health for years. But, I ended up learning so much about myself and have experienced and felt life to the fullest. And the fact is without all my struggles, I wouldn't be the person I am today. That's what makes me special. All of our unique circumstances build us into the people we become. So don't ask for someone else's life. Live yours as if everything is happening on purpose, just the way it was supposed to.

"KEEP YOUR FACE ALWAYS TOWARD THE SUNSHINE AND THE SHADOWS WILL FALL BEHIND YOU"- WALT WHITMAN

Chapter 60

So, on the one hand, one could say I showed myself that no human being is invincible from adversity. But, from another perspective, I could say that I accomplished my goal of becoming bulletproof. I showed myself what I could handle. My body went through hell, but I emerged stronger than ever, both mentally and physically. Maybe I didn't show that I could control everything and prove to be invincible, but I built my body and mind to OVERCOME anything. **What I couldn't prevent, I COULD HANDLE, and that is what makes true strength**. We can't always control what happens to us, but we can most definitely control how we respond. When life hits, we can cower and surrender to the thought that the world doesn't want us to succeed, or we can take it as a challenge to keep fighting and to become the strongest person, adding one piece of armor at a time. So, although my goal was to be 100% healthy and to be this human being who wasn't affected by adversity, I realize now that the adversity made me who I am today. The bulletproofing came from the struggles, and the added life experience has made me a stronger person.

MY DESIRE TO PLEASE
Chapter 61

While writing this book, I learned a lot about myself and why I am the way I am. As James once said to me, "You're not crazy, that's just what makes you Jared." A large part of who I am has come from a desire to make those around me happy. I don't like others being upset with me, especially parents, and I don't like to disappoint. This inadvertently puts a lot of pressure on me. And I have carried this into my friendships; I love to make others happy.

I have always been sensitive from a young age and have had all those feelings amplified in recent years. I think one of the reasons that I have made the effort to be such a good person to others is because I don't want them to feel what I have felt (the bad stuff—even though I know that adversity makes you stronger when you overcome it and learn from it). It's a strange concept, because one might think going through the health struggles and mental challenges would make me cynical or bitter, but the truth is I wish that I can take the brunt of the struggles so that no one close to me ever has to feel that way. Whenever I'm around these kids who I'm influencing, I want them to know that I'm there for them and will not give up on them, where others might. I love it when my parents tell me how proud they are of me. I love it when these kids' parents tell me how much their kids love me or how proud they are of me for accomplishing things, because I inspire them and have such a tremendous influence on their kids. It really means the world to me and lets me know that I'm doing the right thing.

However, you can't please everyone, and some people aren't worth trying to please as I have learned. It's pivotal to make sure that you are doing what you want FOR YOU first and foremost. It is not "selfish" to do what's right for you because as I often say, you can't give to others from an empty cup. First, you have to fill your own cup, and then you will have more to give to others! However, there is also something to be said for having people who count on you and those who you want to make proud and don't want to let down! Yes, it is very difficult to completely ignore others' opinions, especially if you're someone who's sensitive like me. So, I think the key as with many other things is acceptance. It comes down to accepting that there will be negative opinions out there, but these should never affect your perceptions of yourself or your life decisions. Not everyone will agree with everything you say or what you put out into the world, especially when you are speaking hard truths. I'm not saying that what I say is "the ultimate truth" or that I have all the answers and that you have to listen to me, but it is imperative for everyone to seek out the truth for themselves, no matter how uncomfortable it may be. "You can take authority as your truth or you can take truth as authority."- Gerald Massey

Having accountability is a healthy way of looking at your loved ones. Don't let anyone MAKE your decisions and most definitely don't let people who have no importance in your life influence your decisions. At the same time, there is nothing wrong with trying to live up to the healthy standards placed on you by loved ones. If a friend thinks of you as being the nicest person or a role model, then you should try to live up to that. But, just because a family member wants you to play it safe and not try to be a YouTuber, an entrepreneur, a pro athlete or a musician, and rather get a "normal" job, this is a time where you listen to yourself and your ambitions because that is the only way to become your best self. The most surefire way to find your purpose is to follow your passions!

You can't please everyone all the time; your loved ones can be holding you accountable to high standards and serve as motivation when life gets hard. And your doubters will show you what you have to do and are the fuel who can push you to achieve the "impossible." But ultimately the one who must do what's best for yourself is you.

PULLING FROM MULTIPLE SIDES OF MOTIVATION

Chapter 62

One of the initial motivating factors prompting me to work to my limits was actually a pretty common thing for a lot of people, and this idea we will refer to as "haters" or "doubters." Every underdog has had to deal with them. They start off as really annoying and really discouraging, and then you begin to accept them—and then they turn into rocket fuel that gets you jumping out of bed to get better every day and prove these people wrong. Tom Brady will always remember how he was a 6ᵗʰ round draft pick, and Michael Jordan will always remember not being picked for the varsity team in 10ᵗʰ grade. Now, if you ask me, I think a lot of us can relate to far deeper stories about being cut or picked on or not picked for ANY team, but the thing is it still stings them, and these athletes are known as arguably the greatest of all time. It's one major motivation that keeps them hungry. While working to be the best athlete, I took another "seemingly impossible" goal of trying to dunk a basketball. Whenever someone would try to put me down or talk about the idea of something being impossible, it seethed in me. But, with the power of dedication, a strong belief, and hard and smart work, I believe we can achieve far greater than what's currently in front of us. Oftentimes, when people see you trying to better yourself and putting in more work than they would care to do, it makes them mad and they try to pull you back down to their level. One statement that I really can't stand more than just about any other is "It's not like he's going pro" or another one, "People like us can't do that." Don't ever group me into the same category as you because you aren't me. And to me that just sounds like some built in excuses to not give it your all. As I said earlier, maybe you will fail, but maybe you will find out the greatest strength within you that the person standing on the sidelines never could have. I would rather take that chance. As one of my favorite quotes by naturopathic doctor Cassie Huckaby says, "The world has never seen you. How can any book or any person know what you are capable of?" This is why I believe that humans can heal from and overcome anything if they choose to!

Then, over time I began to realize that you need more than one well to pull from. The haters/doubters are like that rocket fuel that will drive you crazy, but you can't only pull from that because that well is often driven by anger and negative emotions, which aren't totally sustainable nor healthy. What you start to realize is that you can't do it all on your own, and over time if you put in that constant work, you'll also gain some supporters and new friends who are hoping for your success. You don't want to let these people down. BOOM: Well number 2 has been formed-- not wanting to let down your supporters and wanting to inspire them and show them how anything is possible. This initially came to me in the form of my campers and the kids who I worked with over the summers and the ones who ultimately became my best friends. These kids believed in me and believed that I was a superhero, so who am I to say they're wrong? When this new motivation came along, I realized that this is a pretty sustainable well to pull from and one that can provide me with consistent fuel and more happiness, since this is fueled by love. Each well has its place.

Another large well to pull from can be the overall purpose and message that you are trying to convey. What is your mission and goal from all this? Because if it's just to prove people wrong, you are doing it for the wrong reasons. My mission was to inspire kids and adults alike, and show them, as well as prove to myself, that anything is possible. Having intrinsic motivation is essential. If you believe you are carrying out a higher calling, such as carrying out this divine path or doing something that will make a huge positive impact, that's some strong stuff to pull from too! It only takes one person to believe this, so that person better be you. Remember that it's not selfish to do things to achieve personal goals and to engage in self-improvement. This is actually the best thing you can do for the world—become the best version of yourself. As Mahatma Gandhi said, "Be the change you wish to see in the world." Chase all your dreams and have no regrets. The world needs more people like this: people who are willing to fail and who can be themselves without fear of being judged, as this inevitably inspires others to do the same.

PATIENCE
Chapter 63

One of the most difficult things to have when it seems like nothing is going right is patience. As Aristotle said, "Patience is bitter but the fruit is sweet." Throughout my healing journey, there was a ridiculous amount of waiting to feel all better. I was doing everything possible—following the right diet (for me), getting sunshine, grounding daily, implementing tons of daily movement inputs, taking all the right supplements and doing a ton of detoxing/opening up my drainage pathways, transforming my life and cutting out the parts I found to be toxic, and using all of my research to get back to 100% health. A lot of it wasn't always comfortable, but I pushed through and told myself to trust the process. Yet, for a long time, it seemed that nothing was changing. This brings me to one of my favorite stories that I looked to: *The Story of the Bamboo Tree.* When a bamboo tree gets planted, at first you see no growth, nothing even happening. Two years go by, three years go by. You continue to water it, and yet still it looks as if there is nothing happening. Four years go by, still nothing. Then, seemingly out of nowhere, after five years of waiting, within a matter of weeks the tree sprouts up into this super tall beautiful tree. How did this happen? During those years where it appeared as if nothing was happening above the surface, below the surface this tree was building its roots, building a strong foundation, putting in the work every day—so that when the time was right, it could blossom.

I view my journeys the same way—my path to health as well as my journeys as an athlete, an influencer/content creator, and as a person. I was constantly watering my roots (and continue to do so), so that when the time was right everything could fall into place and I would be better than ever. Nothing great happens overnight and in my case sometimes you won't see any movement for 5-6-7 years, but that doesn't mean that you are failing or that nothing good is happening. It's just occurring below the surface. Healing takes a long time. Many people didn't truly understand the extent of the damage that was done to my body and thought that maybe I wasn't following the right path by taking the holistic route (which I believe is the only route to true health—taking every aspect of your life and making it your elixir that promotes health and life in all aspects). They doubted that I would ever get better. Some people I couldn't even talk to because I knew they weren't capable of understanding what was required along with the level of patience needed. Thankfully I had my best friends and family members who were my source of encouragement and kept telling me it would get better and that soon I would be there. And of course I had the unwavering belief in myself that full healing was possible! In many ways my athletic journey resembled my healing journey. It was at times frustrating, upsetting, and depressing seeing my desire to perfect everything, yet not achieving the improvements nor receiving the recognition that I was looking for. But, stopping the work wouldn't get me anywhere. Nobody ever arrived at their destination by quitting halfway through. If I were to stop when things got tough, I would have never known my own strength and I wouldn't be here today to write my story. Sticking with it and continuing to grind is what is needed. Almost all of our decisions in life are choosing between short term pain for long term gain, or short term pleasure for long term pain. Even when it seems that nothing is happening, remember that you are working on building a strong foundation and once everything falls into place, then and only then will you be able to blossom. Not many people are able to have that level of patience. If you are able to keep going in spite of the lack of visible progress, you will reap the fruit.

IT'S OKAY TO BE VULNERABLE AND IT'S OKAY TO SHOW WEAKNESS
Chapter 64

We all go through stuff in our lives. And it's a sign of strength to call upon a friend or family member, or in some cases a professional who understands how to empower you, to get us through these things. For instance, when I was at my worst with my speech, there would be times when I couldn't even get out any words, and I would just freeze. I knew exactly what I wanted to say but I just couldn't speak it. And on top of that, when it did come out, it would often be slurred or I would stammer and stutter to make things worse. I became self-conscious around a lot of people. I would try super hard to talk as little as possible to some people. But, when it came to the people in my life who truly made an effort to understand what I was going through and show empathy and compassion, it was amazing how showing my weakness made my bond with these people grow stronger. I knew I could trust these people with anything.

They would encourage me to keep speaking and made it clear that they were interested in what I had to say, and would be patient in listening and would give me the time I needed. These few people made me feel comfortable in my own skin and not self-conscious and actually gave me the strength that I needed to keep pushing. We are all afraid at times to put ourselves out there in the open with no safety net, but sometimes we can gain strength from revealing our weaknesses and being willing to be vulnerable. This makes us stronger and can help turn our weaknesses into strengths. It's like in the movie *Inside Out,* which is an excellent portrayal of how our emotions work and how all are important to making the complete person. "Joy" doesn't realize this at first and just wants Riley to be happy all the time, but then she learns that every time sadness emerged, it ended with a person comforting her and making her feel strong again. Without sadness or weakness, we don't allow ourselves to strengthen and let others come into our lives to make things better. Every emotion and every feeling we have plays a role and has a purpose, whether we like it or not. So, it's important to not suppress or make these

270

feelings go away. Just as with meditation, we don't push away thoughts, and the same applies here. They are there for a reason too and must be felt.

Another example is if you're an athlete and you are right handed and you just continue to hide your left hand for fear of revealing your weakness, eventually there will come a point when you are not reaching your full potential and it will come back to bite you. You have to be willing to miss the shots, even in front of others, in order to work on your weakness and reach your full potential.

It's okay to cry, crying releases pent up negative emotions and does not mean you are a weak person. As the famous quote from Johnny Depp goes, "People cry not because they're weak, but because they've been strong for too long." We can only keep it together for so long, and sometimes we just need to release and allow others to come to our side and get us back to the positive side.

MY ULTRA COMPETITIVE NATURE
Chapter 65

From the moment I started playing sports I have been a super competitive person. I'm one of those people who hates losing even more than I like winning. I've cried from losing "meaningless" games before because I feel that every game I'm playing matters. No matter what it is, whether it be video games, actual sports games, mini golf, or an arcade game, I want to win so badly. This is another component of my work ethic. Because when you want to win so badly, you know that you have to work for it. But, it can also lead to constant comparison to others. This has its benefits and its downsides. It pushes me to always go harder, but it can also contribute to unregulated stress and depression. This is one of the reasons why so many people say to not take social media so seriously. It is inherent in social media that we are going to compare other people's lifestyles to ours. Whether it be one that is more lavish or more fun or whether one's body looks better than ours, or if someone has more followers or gets more likes than we do. This can most definitely lead to depression and social stress.

But, on the positive end of it, it makes me chase the impossible and push myself harder by seeing others doing big things. It's like when someone says that the only way to get faster is to be the slowest person in the race. Even if what I am chasing is "unrealistic," I still believe that by going after that goal I'll get further than I ever would have, had I not had the competition. As easy as it should be to just look at myself and what I'm doing, my anxiety leads me to compare and sometimes I just can't help it. Seeing that other humans are capable of these incredible things, and understanding that I possess the same power within me, is inspiring. It doesn't mean that everything is meant for me though, considering how we also have our own unique gifts that make us special which is important to keep in mind. For instance, just because I believe that we all have limitless potential to be whomever we want and go after any goals, whether it be start a podcast, dunk a basketball, become a musician—it doesn't mean that everything is part of YOUR individual path or purpose.

Having said all that, there is definitely much more merit in comparing yourself to yourself. If you got a tiny bit better from one day to the next, that is still a win. What I have realized having gone through my crazy illness and health recovery journey is that we are all at different places in our lives, and we all have different challenges and different obstacles that we have to overcome. To look at someone else's life or skills and wanting them to be your own is unfair to yourself and doesn't give you the credit that you deserve. Maybe the person you're looking at was born gifted with genetics (that suits them for that specific task), or born into the perfect situation that gave them their skillset, and they are succeeding in spite of their lack of hard work, or maybe they didn't have the challenges that you have had to overcome. But it doesn't mean that you can't reach their level or even surpass their level. It may just take you some more time. For example, when I was trying to dunk and become a better basketball player and stronger in the weight room, even when my health and digestion issues were acting up like crazy, basically sapping me of all my energy and causing me sleepless nights, it was not right of me to expect the same amounts of improvement as someone who didn't have the same stresses on their body. That didn't mean I wasn't going to try just as hard anyway, but it meant I had to be more understanding of what I was going through and expect some setbacks and bad workouts and small improvements. In order to stay sane, I had to give myself self-love and realize that when the time was right I would achieve all my goals. So I had to remain patient for a really long time and consistently do all of the small simple things on a daily basis to restore my health.

One really hard thing to accept is that you can be doing everything "right" with whatever it is that you are trying to achieve—putting in all the work and being smart, yet still this life has zero guarantees. What I like to say is that if you're an underdog especially, you have to do everything right—research the best ways to train/practice, what to eat, and tailor your lifestyle to your goals, or whatever it may be. There is such minimal room for error, but even then there is no knowing how long it will take to achieve your goals; there are no guarantees. But without that work, you have no chance. If everything were guaranteed, there would be no joy in

273

the journey and no falling in love with the process. No getting back up after every failure and going back into the lab to reconfigure. How much fun would it be if you were playing a game that you knew you couldn't lose? After a while, that would get pretty boring. There must be a possibility of agonizing defeat in order to know the thrill of success! That's part of what makes the journey so fulfilling. Also, what I've learned is that oftentimes it's not about win or lose…the joy is in the playing.

WE ALL START SOMEWHERE
Chapter 66

If you're constantly focused on what others are doing and accomplishing, you'll miss the chance to appreciate all of the great things you are doing. Over-comparing can kill your drive. It can stress you out and make you feel like if you don't get to that person's level, then you didn't accomplish anything. Never downgrade yourself or what you are accomplishing by being so impressed with others. We all have different starting points. Understand that as long as you are giving it your all, then what you are doing is amazing. I'm not saying that we should be applauding mediocrity or be happy with participation awards, but we have got to appreciate our best work and our own accomplishments and remember that we all have to start somewhere. The world wants you to always be comparing yourself to others, and I have a lot of trouble with this myself, but we must maintain perspective. What you are doing is important and matters, and don't let anyone change that or get that twisted.

So many people are often allowing themselves to be blown away by what celebrities are doing or what the people who started from the top are doing. And I actually believe this is done purposely by the media to make us see the "people in power" (although power is often an illusion) or these celebrities as being "above" the rest of us, so that we don't realize how amazing we are! There is definitely something to be said when it comes to this "celebrity worship syndrome." This is why I no longer look up to most celebrities outside of the handful of ones who I truly believe are good people and did things the right way. And I definitely don't "idolize" them, especially considering that many of them work for dark occultist agendas (this doesn't mean I can't still be inspired by certain aspects of their journeys or quotes such as the ones used in this book as long as I can use proper discernment, but we do need to be aware of these aspects). I am much more impressed when someone starts from the bottom and makes a huge jump. It takes more courage to stay in it when you aren't the best. But, every jump matters. If you start at the top and don't keep raising your own levels, then I don't really look to you for inspiration.

Let's face it, there are some people out there who are seemingly "born lucky." I don't believe a ton in "pure luck," but when it comes to certain things such as sports or business, there are people who everything just seems to go right for even though they lack the qualities of the "underdog" that I mentioned before. And I have seen a lot of this firsthand. However, due to this lack of what it truly takes, oftentimes they fall into trouble down the road, as a result of not having built up this grit. The same thing goes for content creators who become big right away but then can't sustain it. Indeed the harder you work and the more positive energy you put out into the world and the ether, and the more you speak your goals into existence, the "luckier" you will get. Just because you're a small fish in a big pond doesn't mean that the work you are doing doesn't matter. Keep grinding, and in time you will have others wanting to be like you too.

Jared Weiss

THE BIG QUESTION WHEN IT COMES TO SUCCESS

Chapter 67

People are always asking others—how can I be as successful as you? How can I jump higher? What type of workouts can I do to look like you? How much do I have to study to be as smart as you? Where should I invest to make as much money as you? First off, these questions can never be definitively answered because everything needs to be customized to your needs and stage in life. Often I hear people responding that you have to want it bad enough or that you have to work hard, and both are very true, but are only part of the equation. I believe the most important thing when it comes to success at anything is, how many times are you willing to fail? The reason why people quit and why so many don't believe that anything is possible is because they gave up after the second, third, or fourth try and decided it wasn't gonna happen, it wasn't meant to be for them, and it's time to try something new. The greats have failed thousands and thousands of times before eventually achieving their level of success. One of my favorite song lyrics goes, "The greats weren't great because at birth they could paint, the greats were great because they paint a lot"-Macklemore. I believe that anything is possible as long as you stay in the game long enough. Just because you were cut from the team once or you didn't get accepted into the school of your dreams doesn't mean you were not meant to do what you desire. It just means you have to accumulate more failures in order to succeed. This is hard for a lot of people to hear. Recently I was looking back on an old Facebook post of mine from 2012 where I said how I had just finished up a tough vertical jump workout and would be dunking soon... it took me until 2019 just to touch the rim, and I wouldn't (officially) touch it again until 2024! Do you know how much I went through just to get to that point? Countless workouts, countless failures, countless injuries, and of course a life threatening illness and ensuing health struggles. Where others would have given up after a year, it took me 8 years just to get a piece of the puzzle. When I was healing from my severe health issues and my speech was severely impacted, there was no telling when or if I would ever get back to the way it was. Eight years later and I still wasn't fully healed yet. Or when my digestive issues started and I started my first naturopath program, and two years go by with only minimal, not even really outwardly noticeable improvements. It wasn't time to give up, but rather I needed to do more research and get some more help to find out what else was going on and how to help it along. Healing is a slow steady process that's always moving forward, even through setbacks, but the longer you endure, the more appreciation and respect you have for the process. "Nothing worth having comes easy" is what my phone background has said since 2014. And that's the 100% truth. How much failure are you willing to take before you give up? How many bumps and bruises can you handle before you break? You have got to be in this for the long haul, and if not, you can just quit right now. You may have heard that "you miss 100% of the shots you don't take." Well you may have to take 1000 shots before that 1st shot goes in.

OUTSIDE THE BOX
Chapter 68

There is a need to be skeptical when hearing information. Just because "everyone" believes something doesn't make it true. Often the real experts are the ones called crazy and are the outside the box thinkers. As one of my main people who I follow in the holistic health world, Alec Zeck (who's a supporter of mine as well), often says, don't blindly trust him and don't blindly trust anyone. We all have to do our own research and come to our own conclusions. He often tries to present his own information by asking questions which helps to get his viewers thinking. This is a great way to stimulate healthy skepticism. A lot of people who let their egos get too big start to see themselves through this "God-like complex." They claim to be the ultimate purveyors of truth. So what I've realized is that it's important to learn and take the best aspects from everyone, and then form your own opinions and belief systems and routines that work best for you. As I've learned from Alec, as well as Sam Tripoli's Tin Foil Hat podcast amongst others, a lot of what we've been taught to believe has just been indoctrination and has continually been pushed to us by the mainstream media and the history books as a way of furthering a specific agenda. And the only reason why we believe these things is because we've been told not to question them or we get ridiculed if we do.

As I like to say, the only thing that I'll ever know with 100% certainty is that I will never know anything with 100% certainty. In other words, always be learning. Don't listen to those who act like know it alls, and realize that there is always another level and a deeper dive into learning. Do your own research, find others who have done truly independent unbiased research, get some first-hand experience, and always think critically and for yourself.

When you become obsessed with something, others will often try to tell you that you are crazy or call you weird. Some of the greatest minds have been called those things and it didn't seem to stop them.

The first time I was telling James about how I hadn't eaten anything unhealthy since I was in 8th grade; I told him that's just me being crazy, which is something I often say because I am someone who has very obsessive tendencies. When I do something I go all in on it 1000% or don't go at all. But his profound response resonated once more, "That's not crazy, that's just Jared. It's who you are." That really stuck with me. It was his way of saying that we are all unique, and doing things differently or being different from others doesn't make you crazy, it just makes you you.

Oddly enough, my all-in lifestyle choices often get others very interested. My way of thinking, even if others don't agree with it, can be interesting to those who are open to listen. So, being different can make you interesting too. A lot of times when I would meet someone new, if Jacob was there with me, he would introduce me by saying "This kid hasn't eaten a cookie in 10 years and works out multiple times every day." (LOL) But immediately everyone would be questioning how I do it and start inquiring to know more. That's another thing; just because someone might be very quiet or shy doesn't mean they don't have the most interesting story to tell. Around my friends and family and people who I'm comfortable with, I will talk a lot and love speaking my mind, but around people who I don't feel comfortable with, I can be shy and won't say much (although I have gotten way more comfortable recently speaking to new people as a result of meeting so many people at my gym, as well as doing the podcast with people whom I haven't spoken with prior. I'm actually probably the most confident I've ever been in myself these days). In high school, it was always a topic of conversation that I was trying to dunk a basketball and wanted to try to be a pro-level athlete. And as I said earlier, my "friends" would always tell me that's impossible and to give up and be more like them. Because that was what they wanted to accept. It's just like the story of the crabs in a bucket. If you put a bunch of crabs in a bucket, as soon as one tries to crawl out, the others will immediately attack it and try to pull it back down to where they are. People's egos get threatened when you try to make more of yourself because they have accepted that self-improvement isn't possible. As the character played by Will Smith says in *Pursuit of Happiness*, "People can't do something themselves, they want to tell you you can't do it. If you want something, go get it, period." That's the way I live my life. I will not let others dictate what I do. Whether you like me or not, I am gonna be me.

I DON'T LIKE IT WHEN PEOPLE TELL ME WHAT I "SHOULD" DO WITH MY LIFE

Chapter 69

We all have an obligation to be the best versions of ourselves and to go after greatness. Even if we fall flat on our face, we have to go after it, because without that we will never know what might have been. One of my favorite quotes comes from the movie *Coach Carter*, "Our deepest fear is not that we are inadequate, our deepest fear is that we are powerful beyond measure…Your playing small does not serve the world. There is nothing enlightened about shrinking so that other people won't feel insecure around you. We are all meant to shine as children do…And as we let our own lights shine, we unconsciously give other people permission to do the same. As we are liberated from our own fear, our presence automatically liberates others." Don't play small just to satisfy others who doubt you, instead dream big so that others feel inspired to dream big as well.

Ever since I was in middle school and high school, others from peers to family members have always tried to tell me what I should do with my life and what I should be. But in my view, they were always selling me short because they have no idea what I can and will be capable of. Your world vision for me doesn't satisfy what I want to do. I really don't like it when others tell me what to believe, how to think, and who I should be. This is my life and I'm gonna live it the way I want to. I'm going to learn a ton along the way, and I will constantly be tweaking, but it will be "my way" just as Frank Sinatra said. Let me clarify—I appreciate the suggestions when a friend or family member tells me how great I am at whatever it is and suggests that maybe I would like doing that job. And typically these suggestions are well meaning. But, if you don't even know my goals or the big dreams I have planned for my life and you start mapping out my life for me, I don't want to hear that.

When I try to help others, I allow and encourage them to dream as big as possible because whatever they choose, it will end up being greater than if they had thought small. Moreover, I believe that I have gone through what I have with my severe health challenges in order to prepare me for an extraordinary life and incredible work. I owe it to myself to show that anything is possible. If I overcame and survived and thrived through my struggles, then I must be meant for greater things. If I went through hell and did something that didn't showcase me in the best possible way, I would be undoing God's work of using me as a vessel to inspire others.

Ultimately, I have life size dreams and goals for myself and have plans for accomplishing them, so if you're not gonna support them, then you're just in the way. I don't need that negativity. There was a video posted by Eric Thomas, a motivational speaker; he said that when he tells someone he wants to buy a property, if you're saying, "I don't know about this, it doesn't sound like a good idea and might be hard to pay for it"…he doesn't need that. He says that when he has an idea to do something big, he needs his circle to be like, "Yeah let's gooo!!!" If I respect you and your opinions and I understand how highly you think of me and you understand what my goals are, then by all means suggest away, and I will love you for it and listen to you. But, any decision I make will be my own.

THE BIG MISTAKE THAT I ALONG WITH MANY OTHERS HAVE MADE

Chapter 70

When you work so hard to achieve something it becomes easy to tie your identity into how good you are at that thing. But truthfully if you always tie your identity into things you have no "direct" control over and things that are tied into others' opinions, you will often be disappointed. Your identity should not be tied into what you do, but rather who you are. You can certainly control becoming a better and a nicer person, and you can always control how much effort you put into your craft. For the longest time (and I still struggle with this a bit today), I've allowed a part of myself to be defined by how good I am at basketball and how good of an athlete I am. When you have coaches who are as hard on you as mine were on me, and when you get criticized to the point of tears every time you play a bad game and you get showered with praise every time you play a great game, you start to think that is who you are. I understand that many coaches just want the best for you, but I always felt like there should have been more of a focus on my work ethic leading up to the game and my effort going into the game because, of course I always wanted to play well!

Moreover, my "friends" early on would be tied into this too. If I was playing really well I would seemingly have more friends and people wanting to be around me, but as soon as things went downhill that seemed to change. These are what we call fair-weather friends. You need friends who are there for you through sickness and health, through the games when you're not scoring and the games when you're scoring a bunch. That's the test of a true friend. Know who is around you, and keep an eye on who leaves if things go downhill. After having been through tremendous uphill battles with my health, I wanted to be defined by my fight and how I overcame everything, and use what I went through to inspire others. As Brooke Shields recently said, "How you respond is going to define you. Adversity won't make you as much as it will reveal you because you see who you are. You see what you're made up of." I was always thought of as the nicest person to a lot of my peers, and now I realize how that will almost always be more important than what I do as an athlete or a writer or an influencer or anything. Of course I will always try to be the best at everything I do, but I'm still learning that those things don't define me. I love being an athlete and that is a huge part of my life, but I can't control others' opinions of me. I have my effort and my determination and who I am as a person, and no one can take that away from me.

You have to understand that you are more than your stats and more than your grades or your profession—you are above all a person who has principles and a brand with a message that you are showcasing at all times. What do you most want to be remembered for?

Understanding what's really important helps put things in perspective. Not getting an A on a test or not having a great game might matter a lot in the moment and I'm not saying it shouldn't, but everything needs perspective. Of course these things can hurt. Or maybe you're in high school and you feel like if you aren't popular or if a certain person doesn't like you, your life is over. Sometimes it takes a severe health issue or a difficult life challenge to give you this perspective, or sometimes you just have a good grasp of life. When you're in that hospital bed, do you really think it matters what others thought of you in high school? That's not getting you that next breath. The more you understand the importance of perspective, the better you play and perform. When you tell yourself (and I know from experience) that if you miss this shot your coach might take you out, or your teammates may turn on you, or your peers might not consider you to be a good player and then you won't play in college, this is a ridiculous amount of pressure to put on yourself. This can make you tense up because you are worrying about things you can't directly control, and you are placing too much importance on this game and this shot. Being passionate and caring about your craft is an incredible thing that I pride myself on. But when you get away from why you fell in love with that craft in the first place, and it starts causing more stress and pressure than it is giving you joy and fun, you start to lose yourself and it becomes like a job. Same goes for me as a content creator. I constantly reiterate to myself and others that the impact I make will always be more important than the number of likes or views. Those things can be an awesome reward, but as long as I positively impact one life and I'm proud of my message and my work, it's worth it to me!

Being someone who has dealt with tons of anxiety and just being a very sensitive kid makes it tough to have fun sometimes with the things I want to be great at. That's why I need to constantly remind myself of why I fell in love with these things in the first place. And now I have this newfound perspective, so it's like does this game or test really matter in the grand scheme of things? Our ego and our mind will sometimes try to make us forget this. I'm not one of those people who believes we have to "kill the ego." Our egos do have their place and are not only bad as some make it seem. But, the more present you are able to be when you can just enjoy every moment and control what you can and place more importance on your effort, being an amazing person, and your health and happiness—the better your game and life will get too, because you will be loose and allow your skills to flourish. Sometimes it helps to think back to when you first started practicing your craft. The first time you picked up a basketball and started shooting around and couldn't make a shot or even come close to the rim, but you were smiling and laughing and running around anyway as if you had won the championship. Or maybe you want to do well on a test, so you think back to the time when everyone first considered you smart. Maybe your parents had you doing math problems in front of family friends and you loved showing this skill off. As a content creator, maybe you think back to that post you made where someone told you it was exactly what they needed to hear. That is one of the many reasons why I love being around kids. They can teach us so much about gratitude for every moment. Get back to why you began working on your craft: because it was fun for you and you genuinely enjoy getting better, and that will remove a lot of the pressure and the stress of the situation. I really wish I would've understood this a long time ago, but there's no better place to start than now.

This is also why Ryan Fitzpatrick, the Harvard grad and journeyman quarterback, is one of my favorite athletes of all time. On every team he played for, he was basically playing on borrowed time. He was never the "quarterback of the future" or the one who the team was counting on to win games. But, if you ever watched him, you could tell that everyone loved playing with him. You can see the enjoyment he got from playing football and how he lived in the moment. He genuinely loved playing the game and looked like a little kid having fun out there. He would have press conferences wearing gold chains or showing his beard and chest hair. He didn't worry about what others thought of him. And this love of the game got him to set NFL records that some of the "greatest of all time" could never even dream of achieving.

UNDERDOG
Chapter 71

Throughout most of my life I have viewed myself as an underdog. I often felt that I had to work harder than everyone else for everything that I accomplished. However, whenever I achieve, the glory feels that much greater. As Nate Robinson says in his book *Heart Over Height*, "I was given a lot of heart but no height. I'll take that any day." He was one of the smallest players to play in the NBA but he was ferocious on the court. As soon as I saw him, I thought maybe that could be me. People would say to me, "That's just genetics" or "He's one in a million," but I didn't care. Seeing one person do what I wanted to do was enough to show me that maybe it was possible. Nate was a 3 time slam dunk contest champion at 5'9! My grandpa and I used to love watching him. And even more, he was a dominant 2 sport athlete as he excelled at football too. Yeah maybe if I was given more natural abilities and was taller, maybe I would be a better athlete. But I never looked at it like that. I love putting in the time and working on things that I love. It feeds my hunger and allows me to keep going when things get tough. I have always had this insatiable desire to be great at everything I do. It's just the way I was built. I don't take no for an answer and I don't allow others to tell me what's possible and what isn't. Those who landed at the top of the mountain will never know what it's like to have to work for everything. Every tiny gain seems like it takes a lifetime to earn, but it is always well worth it. This 100% was what guided me through my healing journey as well. If healing weren't so difficult, you wouldn't value it as much and wouldn't have this appreciation for the body's capability to do it. This is what I preach to my friends and those who I try to inspire: You don't need conditions to be great, and you don't need perfect circumstances in order to keep going and keep grinding. There will be setbacks and times where it feels like giving up is the only option, but the only way out is through. When it feels like you're running in place or can't find the way out, remember that it will get better, but you can't give up. This is the mentality of the underdog. We fight until we can't anymore!

One super fascinating thing I heard recently from famous basketball skills trainer and performance coach Paul James Fabritz aka PJF

Performance, is that a lot of pro players make it to the NBA in spite of their training and not because of it. So many of them were born with natural skills and natural athleticism, and in fact have very poor diets and really lack proper training. I have seen a lot of this first hand when I was playing AAU and also from listening to top athletes discuss their training regimens. Sometimes it's crazy to fathom all of the work I have put in and the ridiculous amounts of research and trial and error I have done just to get to where I am, when some people don't have to do any of it. When I was going through my digestive ailments and all of my treatment methods even though I had eaten only what I considered to be "healthy foods" since 8th grade, it almost seemed unfair because others could seemingly eat whatever they wanted without issues (even though an unhealthy lifestyle will likely catch up to them at some point). But the truth is, it gave me a chance to fall in love with my body and myself, and I wouldn't have it happen any other way. This was how it was meant to be. I love working hard. I love learning new things. It excites me. And when I see something that I'm not good at, I view it as an opportunity for growth. Be careful who you're taking the advice from. Look for people who had to go into the trenches themselves and had to grind for every last drop. These will usually be the ones who are best able to guide you to where you want to go.

WHEN SOMETHING BAD HAPPENS YOU HAVE THREE CHOICES. YOU CAN EITHER LET IT DEFINE YOU, LET IT DESTROY YOU OR LET IT STRENGTHEN YOU.

Chapter 72

There is always a choice to make. Maybe it's not the first option or the second option or what you were expecting, but you do have at least somewhat of a say in what goes on with your life, which is where free will comes in. Circumstances don't have to define us. If we make the best of things and try to turn a negative into a positive, then we can allow that situation to strengthen us. Being bitter or giving up doesn't do any good for anyone. In one of my favorite books *The Stuff* by Sharlee Jeter and Sampson Davis, Sharlee mentions how when a vase breaks, you can try to put it back together the same way, throw it out, or put it back together in a new way with a new form that looks even better. This was very powerful. Putting it back together the same way will probably not work, and throwing it out is the equivalent of giving up on it altogether. But if you have the grit and determination, you can see potential in creating something new that could be better than the initial vase. Maybe you didn't get picked for the job you wanted or got cut from the team that you worked so hard to make. It will take time to get over it, and you have to allow yourself the time to feel sad so that that emotion can pass through you. But after that, if you continue to act like things are always gonna be bad and it's time to stop trying, you let that circumstance win. No matter what it is, you can always create something different and better than the original as long as you have the growth mindset. Remember that nothing is permanent and the bad times won't last forever, so it's up to you to adopt that mindset. "When life gives you lemons, make apple juice and leave everyone wondering how you did it."

When we workout, we are breaking down muscle to ultimately build it back up stronger than before. It's the same thing when it comes to our emotional and mental health and becoming a stronger person with a stronger mindset. We must first accept that which cannot be controlled, and then we make the comeback to emerging stronger than ever before. Our hearts can't grow unless we give it the right tools to build back up; just as after a workout if we want to build muscle we need a healthy protein source. Think of things such as a never give up attitude, a willingness to start up again, gratitude, a great support team, and a belief in something greater than yourself as these tools.

BELIEVE IN YOURSELF BEFORE OTHERS DO

Chapter 73

You have to act and look the part before you ever get the part. If you're trying to be a smarter person/student, start studying and researching how a truly smart person would, and work on critical thinking. Think and believe that you're already smart, and in time your brain will rewire to level up and become what you consistently do. Be strong with your intentions. I once heard someone say, "You don't rise to the occasion, you fall to your level of preparation." To become a top level athlete you don't just start by saying I'm gonna be a top level athlete. Think to yourself how would a top athlete train, how much would a top athlete sleep, what types of foods does a pro athlete eat, would a high level athlete be upset after missing a shot or would they be willing to take that shot again and again? Even if your guidelines might be stricter than that type of person actually is, you will be setting yourself up for great things to come. In a recent podcast with David Parker, Dawn Lester, and Alec Zeck, one of the most powerful parts was when David said, "Stop desiring and start expecting." This is how you create and manifest your life and essentially build heaven on earth.

There will always be detractors and people trying to make you scared of pursuing your goals, or my least favorite thing to hear is to "be realistic." During my high school sports career I always dreamed of playing college sports. My coach made fun of me by calling me "D1," and all the other kids told me it was never gonna happen and that it was impossible. But, I trained harder than anyone in the world, I followed a super strict diet, and made tons of sacrifices (even though I wasn't perfect with what I was sacrificing as I mentioned earlier). I continued working on my game even when others said I was wasting my time. I went to numerous college camps, made highlight tapes and sent them out, and in spite of all that doubt and not being this "highly recruited" athlete, I received my D3 offers and came within inches of walking on to Cornell basketball. I also had a D3 track offer and soccer interest too. How did I do that? Because I saw in myself what others refused to see in me. A lot of things didn't go the way I had planned. I received a lot of rejection and disappointment along the way, but I continued to hustle. Others would have said it was a waste of time and money to keep pursuing those goals. But I had a lot to prove to myself. I was betting on myself. And today because of all the doubt I've faced and my refusal to give up, I'm miles better than I was in high school, and this attitude has translated into all aspects of my life as I have evolved as a human being. I always visualized myself as being the best me at whatever I did. The same thing happened with my dunk journey. I saw it before others had any faith in me. Sometimes you do have to walk the journey alone, but as long as you believe you can do it, go after it with all you've got. If you fail, you fail, but always go down swinging.

When peers told me that I wasn't smart enough to get into an Ivy League school, I didn't say okay, you know what, you're right. Instead I put my head in the books and studied my butt off. And when they still said I couldn't get into those schools I applied to every one and got rejected by every one except for one, but I still did it...one is all it takes. I am not saying any of this stuff to brag at all. I could just as easily tell you all of the times I tried and failed. But, the point I want to get across is that you can't let others decide the path for you. You pave your own way and keep trying again and again. You have to see the vision. If you see it one way, don't allow others who settle for mediocre detract you. And even if you don't reach your desired goals—I mean I "failed" too many times to count on my goals as you've read—I can say with certainty that I got much further in everything had I not tried at all. Others will often tell you to be more "realistic." Being "realistic" usually gets you to accept what others believe is possible. But, what if there was so much more that you could do if only you saw your limitless potential? What is the reason why others tell you to be realistic? So that they don't have to chase goals and put in the work because they don't think it's possible. This justifies their own limited worldview and oftentimes laziness for themselves. Well they aren't you. There may be a one in a million chance of my dream coming true, but I say I'll take those odds as long as that one is me. This is how you become great. The greats let their fires burn brighter than any doubter or hater said they could. You may have to get rid of some people from your life who don't share your vision. I remember every word that the

293

people who doubted me and tried to bring me down said. But, now I can thank those people because they showed me what I had to do. I found outlets to turn the pain into gains and thrived on this energy. And once I started finding the right people who actually supported and encouraged me, I had motivation in all directions to pull from. I had both positive and negative energy—the yin and the yang could help me to make progress far greater than what was "realistic." And interestingly enough, the more I started to focus my own attention and energy on the more positive people and positive energy in my life, the more support I've been able to garner!

Every person who's ever achieved a great challenge has been somewhat "delusional" at one point or another. And this may sound like bad advice, but I think that's what it takes. You have to be willing to see what you can be rather than what you are right now. Maybe you are not a skilled athlete right now, or you are not the smartest student, or aren't very competent at your job, but if you start seeing yourself as capable of being the best, you will start making significant improvements. If I would have listened when the doctors told my family that I might not make it or that I would never be able to speak right again, where would I be today? To sum it all up, you can either settle for mediocre and keep telling yourself the lie that you weren't meant to do great things, or you can chase the impossible and at the very least land amongst the clouds. The choice is yours.

When former pro football player turned baseball player, Tim Tebow, was asked about what it would be like trying to play a new sport professionally, he had this response, "People will say 'what if you fail? What if you don't make it?' Guess what? I don't have to live with that regret. I would rather be someone who can live with peace and no regret than being so scared I didn't make the effort."

"CLICK"-DON'T FAST FORWARD THROUGH LIFE. THERE IS MUCH GOOD TO BE FOUND WITHIN THE 'BAD'

Chapter 74

As the movie, *Click*, shows us, you should not fast forward your life or be living on autopilot. There is much to be learned during times when life knocks you down. There is often much more good going on in our lives than we realize. I have always tried to be an optimist and maintain my positive happy outlook on life. And most of the time I've succeeded. However, having gone through everything with my health, it was definitely impossible to always be happy every second and I think that's understandable, yet every day I would wake up with hope that today was gonna be the day I felt better. Imagine doing that for over 9 years. There were times when I would fake a smile or tell people that I was good and everything was going well, even when this was far from the truth. But also, many of my best times with friends and family and some of my most incredible accomplishments and favorite moments came during those years when I was going through my healing process. This is because I was open to appreciating them. I was looking for the little things to make me happy and I found them. Sometimes I get asked the question: "Do you wish things happened differently with your life?" And the answer is a resounding no—I love my life, through all the ups and downs and the bad times and the good; there's no such thing as a life that's better than yours. As Jake Moscato said when I went on his podcast, "Nothing happened the way it shouldn't have for you…from the doctor who messed you up…to being in the coma and taking the long healing journey with holistic health…everything happened exactly the way it was supposed to!"

The journey can be hard and you might not want to get up and go through the dirty work all the time day after day, but if you live on "autopilot," you're gonna miss all the amazing little things that happen along the way. If I would have just sat in my house everyday waiting till I was 100% healed, I would have been missing out on life. I wouldn't have had my times of overcoming and thriving in spite of adversity. I wouldn't have had my unbelievable times with friends. If I would've waited to talk until my speech was all better, I wouldn't have seen how compassionate and caring my loved ones really are and wouldn't have truly felt the struggle. You have to fully feel the struggles and the negative emotions in order to appreciate the great ones—you have to feel in order to heal.

SOMETIMES IT'S JUST ENOUGH TO PROVE TO YOURSELF THAT YOU DID SOMETHING THAT MATTERS

Chapter 75

The only person who you really have to prove yourself to is you. It's easy to get caught up in trying to prove that you are worthy to others so that they think higher of you. Or sometimes we ONLY work hard to prove our doubters and haters wrong, as I have been guilty of at times. Sometimes we try so hard to prove ourselves to our peers or to society that we matter and that we are doing something great. We try so hard to prove ourselves to colleges or coaches or our followers because this satisfies our ego (which as I mentioned earlier, the ego isn't always a bad thing; it does have its place). But, the more you do things for the wrong reasons, the one who gets hurt is you. The only person who you should worry about proving your worth to is you. We definitely need external motivation at times to drive us further than we would on our own, but never lose sight of why you are doing what you are. When you give something your all, it should be because it makes you happy and it is what you love to do. If you get to the top of something and you realize that you only did it for clout or to please others, it won't feel right. A great quote by Francis Chan is, "Our greatest fear should not be of failure but of succeeding at things in life that don't really matter." Make sure the standard that you are holding yourself to is yours and not society's standards of success. For instance, when I first set out to get into an Ivy League school and to play college basketball, of course I had motivation from people telling me what I couldn't do, but I most importantly wanted to prove to myself how far I could get with my crazy work ethic. However, at times, the reason I would overwork or overtrain and under sleep was because of others' expectations. I was trying to live up to this impossible standard, and I would be the one paying for it by either getting sick or injured or not performing my best due to letting my ego get the best of me.

When I was accepted into Cornell, I realized that I accomplished what I had set out to do. Furthermore, I got the few D3 sports offers/looks when everyone said I was too small to be an athlete. Maybe I didn't ever play college basketball or graduate from an Ivy League school, but proving to MYSELF what I could do was enough. And truthfully, looking back, did I even really need that external validation at all to explain my belief in myself and why I was doing what I was? Probably not. Moreover, if I would've gone back to Cornell while I was still in the midst of chaos during my initial illness recovery, I would've been doing it for the wrong reasons--to show OTHERS that I could graduate from an Ivy League school. When it came to my college basketball tryouts at both Cornell and NYU, when I played some of the best basketball I ever have and proved to myself and everyone else there that I could hang with those guys and excel, the rest was out of my control. It was enough to show MYSELF what I was capable of achieving on the court as an underdog. After some time struggling through my recovery, I wanted to prove to myself and my inner circle of supporters that I was capable of reaching a higher level than ever before. In 2019 when I was working on my skills and shooting baskets at my gym (Lifetime), a pro player from Peru approached me to play 1 v 1 with him after being blown away by my shooting display and ball handling skills during my workout. We were tied up 3-3 in a game to 7, and I believe he won 7-5 or 7-4—but he said to me that I am the first person he had played against who was as quick as he was and said that if I had shot the way I had been shooting before our game, I definitely would have won (in my defense we were using a different ball, but no excuses lol). Afterwards we got into talking and he told me that if I kept working on my game, he believed I should try to look into playing ball overseas, and he encouraged me. There were also numerous times throughout the past few years where I'd be playing pickup ball or a men's league with my brother who plays at RIT, or my friends James, Jake and Corey, and no one knew what I had been through or what was going on inside of me, yet I still had moments where I blew people away with my skills. One time when I was at Lifetime, a bunch of high school and college kids were lining up to watch me and my brother play and we absolutely killed it. One of my friends was watching and said that everyone couldn't stop talking about the kid in the blue shirt (me) as I was on fire. Whether you think I'm good, if you don't think I'm good, it doesn't really matter. All I know is that I have proven a lot to myself. I have achieved many things that others told me was impossible for someone like me. I have also accomplished things that the younger me would be proud of, and that means something!

There's a very powerful scene in the movie *Moneyball* where the baseball team's GM, Billy Beane, is upset after losing in the playoffs despite having changed everyone's beliefs on how a team could win. Billy's assistant, Pete, shows him a video from their minor league club where the catcher's biggest fear was running to 2nd base. The catcher hits the ball, runs past first base and trips. His biggest fear had come true—everyone was laughing at him. What he didn't realize was the ball had gone over the fence; he hit a homerun without even realizing it! This was meant to be a metaphor which I have taken into my own life, especially being someone who can be overly hard on myself and holds myself to a super high standard. When we become overly focused on just the end goal, whether it be feeling 100% better, dunking a basketball, playing college/pro ball, gaining a huge following on social media, or finishing writing this book, we end up missing all of the home runs we're hitting along the way. And even if we don't achieve all of our massive goals that we think we're supposed to, sometimes we end up achieving far greater!

As I said earlier, I struggled at times with separating my worth as a person from my athletics. But as I like to tell those in my inner circle, it doesn't matter to me how good of an athlete you are or how much money you make or how many followers you have or how great of a job you have, it matters to me that you try your best and that you are a good person because that will get you farther than anything else. There's a great quote from the movie *Rudy* where the janitor says to this college football walk-on, "In this lifetime you don't have to prove nothing to nobody except yourself. And after what you've gone through, if you haven't done that by now, it ain't never gonna happen." Fortune noted that Rudy was a little over 5 feet tall, didn't have much athletic ability, yet was able to hang in with the best college football team in the country just based on pure heart. So he had already proved what he could accomplish.

BE THE REASON
Chapter 76

Things might not be going well for you right now. But if you keep pushing onward and never give up, you can one day be the reason that someone else doesn't give up. Be the reason someone smiles because you smiled at them, or maybe you made their day by making them feel appreciated. You can be the "medicine" that someone needed that day. You can show someone they matter. It can even be as simple as sitting with the kid at the lunch table who is sitting all alone. Maybe you see someone having a rough day and you tell them it's all gonna be okay, you know from your own experience. Be the reason someone feels loved. There are a lot of people who need more love; you can give love because it doesn't cost anything. It's 100% free to give a hug or to help someone in their time of need. Be the reason someone believes in the goodness of people by showing them that you are a good person. Treat a friend to lunch for no reason other than to show them how much they mean to you. Offer a helping hand to a loved one. It can be very valuable. Be the reason someone doesn't give up on themselves or their dreams. By showing others your story and explaining how many times you failed before becoming successful, as well as all the difficulties and disappointments you had to encounter before arriving at your goal, maybe you can get others to believe that their life and their dreams aren't over. Maybe they just have to stick with it and by reading or hearing your story, that was enough to keep them going. That's what I think is so amazing about everything I have been through. I think it really gives me so much more understanding of people in general and when they are going through tough times, I feel like I may be able to ease the pain because I know what it feels like. You can never truly understand what someone is going through, but if you let them know that you are there for them, that is often enough to make the person feel your support and they will appreciate it. And oftentimes the favor gets repaid in huge amounts. The more you give, the more you get. That's why it feels so great to help others, because in doing so, your own endorphins emerge as well. I absolutely love it when a close friend or sometimes someone who I haven't spoken to in years will reach out to me on Facebook or

Instagram. They leave a comment and tell me how a post I made was just what they needed to hear or see, because they related their own story to it and they decided to not give up. Sometimes it even brings me to tears. And on the other side of the spectrum, it truly means the world to me when someone, whether my best friend or even a complete stranger, reaches out to me to encourage me to keep going. They show me the strength that I didn't realize I had or tell me how much I mean to them. I often look back to these messages when I need a bit of inspiration.

In one of my favorite songs, "Give Love," by one of my favorite artists, Andy Grammer, he says, "In the end the love we take's got nothing on the love we make so give love." This perfectly describes how we all have so much extra love to give to others and it doesn't run out. The amount of love we have to give only multiplies the more we give it out. The world runs on love!

"YESTERDAY IS HISTORY, TOMORROW IS A MYSTERY, BUT TODAY IS A GIFT. THAT'S WHY WE CALL IT THE PRESENT"

Chapter 77

If there is one thing that I think everyone in the world should do no matter how young or old you are, it's the practice of meditation. I first tried meditation at the age of 15 after learning about it in one of my online basketball training programs. The guy spoke of all of the incredible benefits of meditation, and being someone who always had trouble with anxiety and over-analyzing my thoughts, I thought this would be great to try, and I did have some success with it. Later on at the age of 18, I started to become more serious about it due to the advice of my psychologist and my speech therapist at that time. There are many different ways to meditate. You can repeat a few relaxing or positive words over and over again in your head, you can listen to a guided meditation tape on YouTube, you can do a body scan, or you can just focus on your breath and allow your thoughts to pass through you. You can also use different breathing tempos to get yourself to relax.

The way that I currently do it is I will sit down in a comfortable position and think about the breath passing in and out of me and will repeat a calming mantra to myself, while trying to relax every muscle. And every time a thought or feeling/emotion tries to throw me off course, I will allow it to pass through me and then will gently try to bring my thoughts back to my breath or my mantra, while trying my best not to create resistance towards the thought. I also like to add in some positive visualization, as well as some relaxing music occasionally. Plus, if you still don't think you can do it on your own, there are plenty of awesome guided meditations on YouTube and Spotify.

When I first learned about meditation, I thought this was a way to actually control my thoughts. I thought maybe I could stop some thoughts from coming in and try to bring other "better" thoughts in. The best advice when it comes to meditation is to sit with your eyes closed for as long as you choose, but don't "expect" any benefits. The key to meditation is "don't try," just be. You cannot truly experience peace until you learn to let go and allow your thoughts to be as they please without attacking them. There is this vicious cycle that has occurred numerous times for me which is when a bad thought comes in, you start to obsess over that thought and try to make it go away, and the more you realize that you are thinking about it, the harder you try to push it away and the larger it becomes. This is essentially how anxiety and depression snowball. You need to learn how to let go and allow your thoughts to be. This is not a cure or a medical procedure, but it definitely helps create a space between your thoughts and emotions, and between your thoughts and actions. At first I would meditate once every few days and then sometimes only when I felt up to it. Sometimes you just get too caught up in life that you don't even take a few minutes to yourself. As I learned more and more about myself and as I became more in tune with my spiritual nature, I understood the importance of consistent meditation. Meditation has helped me in so many ways—I truly feel that if more people meditated, we would be able to make better decisions from a clearer mind and just respond to situations, rather than reacting forcefully to everything that gets thrown at us. We would be able to speak from less of an emotional place and more from a calm place where we see what's actually going on. Not only is it important to practice meditation, but it's also essential to truly live it and incorporate the aspects of it as you go throughout your day. I now try to do a 5-10 minute meditation practice 1-2 times daily. I have also read numerous books about meditation and the power of presence and have done research on how super successful people in their fields use meditation.

The ability to be present is truly a superpower. Meditation teaches us how to be present. If any of you watched Michael Jordan's *The Last Dance* docuseries, during the last episode, one of the interviewees said that it was not Michael's supreme athleticism or his skills that made him as great as he was but rather his ability to always be present. I think this speaks volumes, especially because as I read about Phil Jackson and George Mumford, (Phil being his coach and Mumford being the meditation expert who Jackson hired to help bring the team together) both preached meditation to the Bulls championship teams. In addition, Kobe Bryant has many interviews and books which mention his meditation practice, and he has spoken in great depth how what made him so great was his ability to always be present no matter what was going on. He once said, "It's not about how much practice you are doing, but how much of that practice are you PRESENT for that matters."

Surrender the outcome

Being a perfectionist is not easy. There have been many occasions where I tried too hard to make everything perfect and in turn didn't get the results I wanted. Being mindful and practicing meditation and being present can help with this. When you try too hard to do something, you end up losing it. Just like if you were holding a potato chip and you squeezed it too hard you end up breaking it—if you try too hard to achieve a result you can end up with the opposite. The harder you try to get someone to like you, the more they will feel uneasy and not like you. The harder you try to force someone to believe the same thing as you, the more likely they are to be repulsed and turn the other way. The harder you try to perfect your aim on a shot in basketball or baseball or anything, the more often you overthink it and the ball gets gripped too tightly. It's not easy, especially for me, but we have to learn how to surrender the outcome. Sometimes you need to get out of your own way. After you put in all of the work, it's essential to let go and realize that you did everything you could, and now you have to trust your preparation. The way that we perform our best is by letting go of the expectations and our thoughts and trying too hard, and instead focus on just doing and being. Of course you want to do well, and of course you want others to see your greatness, but you need to have faith in your preparation. There is no guarantee that you will do your best or that you will make the team or land the job or get a good grade on the test, but you have to be willing to surrender the outcome and say that whatever happens happens; I know that I gave it my all.

Jared Weiss

DON'T ALLOW WHAT OTHERS ARE DOING GET IN THE WAY OF WHAT YOU'RE DOING

Chapter 78

People often get so caught up in what others are doing and become so impressed with them and then end up feeling like they could never accomplish the same feats. The potential for self improvement gets forgotten way too often. They think these other people have some special gifts that they lack. These people lose sight of their own goals and forget that their life is still going on. Whether seeing people on social media or going to games and events and watching people do impressive stuff, what you don't realize is that that person had to start somewhere, and maybe that's right where you are right now. So many times when I was in high school, I would watch a video of someone dunking, and then I would talk about how great it would be to do the same thing. Then I would actually start attacking the process. This was rare I discovered. Most people would rather passively watch someone do something and talk about how great it is, and then say how they could never do that and why you can't either because you weren't born with their natural talents and gifts. Me, being the believer that anything is possible, I always said maybe that is the case, but if I don't try I'll never know. The world hasn't seen your unique self yet! How could any person or book decide what you can or can't do yet? In other words, you are not just another data point or statistic, so therefore, anything is possible for you. Others would try to stop me and tell me that it was stupid to try, because this was a way of protecting themselves and giving them a reason why they shouldn't try. Let me close out this chapter with a poem that gives me the chills whenever I read it— I first saw this posted by a pro dunker who I follow named Jonathon Clark (aka @jclarkthejumper)…

It Couldn't Be Done
BY EDGAR ALBERT GUEST
Somebody said that it couldn't be done
But he with a chuckle replied
That "maybe it couldn't," but he would be one

Fight Through It

Who wouldn't say so till he'd tried.
So he buckled right in with the trace of a grin
On his face. If he worried he hid it.
He started to sing as he tackled the thing
That couldn't be done, and he did it!

Somebody scoffed: "Oh, you'll never do that;
At least no one ever has done it;"
But he took off his coat and he took off his hat
And the first thing we knew he'd begun it.
With a lift of his chin and a bit of a grin,
Without any doubting or quiddit,
He started to sing as he tackled the thing
That couldn't be done, and he did it.

There are thousands to tell you it cannot be done,
There are thousands to prophesy failure,
There are thousands to point out to you one by one,
The dangers that wait to assail you.
But just buckle in with a bit of a grin,
Just take off your coat and go to it;
Just start in to sing as you tackle the thing
That "cannot be done," and you'll do it.

"FEEL THE FEAR AND DO IT ANYWAY"
Chapter 79

"It's okay to lose to opponent. It's never okay to lose to fear."-Mr. Miyagi

One of the most important life lessons I've heard is to "feel the fear and do it anyway." I first learned this through basketball trainer Taylor Allan. If you know that something is going to be good for you and you want to go through with it, as scared as you may be and as much anxiety as it causes, sometimes you just have to acknowledge that the fear is there, but you can take back control of the wheel from the fear by doing it anyway. When I started doing this, I realized how much more I was saying yes to life. If you want to do something great you have to jump. And that parachute might not open that first time but in order to see what you're truly capable of, you have to take the leap. If I would've listened to my fear all the time, I wouldn't have attempted anything that I have in my life to this point. Being someone who sometimes feels heightened anxiety, it would be easy to say, "You know what, I'm just not gonna try."

I'm not telling you to ignore the fear or to push it away because this was my instinct at first, but as I learned, that just gives power to the fear and makes it grow more. What you need to do is acknowledge that the fear is there. Then say to yourself that it's okay to be scared and it's okay to feel your emotions, as I mentioned earlier, but I'm gonna do this anyway because in the end I'll be happier that I tried it. When I was working at the day camp, there used to be all these special events where counselors had the chance to get up in front of the camp and participate, whether it was counselor makeover day, "American Idol" singing competition, lip sync battle, wrestle mania, or Simon sez competition. And in my early years as a camper and later on as a counselor, I would never want to go up and do these events. I feared being made fun of while having everyone watching me perform in front of the whole camp. It wasn't until the summer of 2014 and onward (after I went through my life-threatening situation and during the years of healing) that I decided I was gonna feel the fear and do it anyway and made it a point to participate in as many events as possible. I would even speak into the microphone as scared as I was with my speech issues, and I participated in every one of those competitions. And I hope that in doing so I inspired others to do the same. It's better to make a fool out of yourself and have a good laugh than to be the one who never tried. In 2015, just months after being out of the hospital, I was made over by my group into the Hulk and was popping my pecs in front of hundreds of people. I was making it a point to show everyone that I wasn't going to let fear control my life.

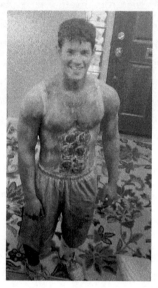

When I was in middle school, I remember watching at one of my older brother's battle of the bands concerts as one high school kid got up on stage and rapped "Hey Mama" by Kanye West, and I was in such amazement at how this kid had so much confidence and was able to get on stage and rap. I thought to myself I don't think I would ever be able to do that. In 2017, I was able to conquer this fear as I performed as Kanye Weiss at camp and did the lip sync to "Heartless." (Recently I actually brought this character back and rapped a song to introduce a new video of mine as well!) Later on that summer, I had a chance to actually sing/rap "T-Shirt" by Migos in the "American Idol" event with two other counselors. The performance didn't go as planned as the music was played too low for any of us to hear—one counselor sang on a toy microphone, and the staff member in charge only let us go for 1 minute.

It didn't sound the way we had practiced it. As I walked off the stage a bit disappointed, a camper comes up to me, maybe he was 6 or 7 years old, and he tells me how amazing he thought I was. Other campers told me how cool they thought our performance was. This was not a waste after all. My whole outlook turned; I may have helped inspire these kids to get up on stage and conquer their fears, and maybe I gave them confidence to go out and do something that they were afraid to do.

Moreover, one of these summers I even asked out a girl on a date and she said yes, although it didn't end up happening (for other reasons). But I did something that I never had done in the past. Also, going back to what I spoke about earlier in this book, I tried out for all these college sports teams. Was I scared when I did all these things? Of course I was! I'm not denying that it was hard, but the more you do it, the more you realize that the fear is all in your head because what is the worst thing that could happen? Everybody laughs at me…the girl says no…I don't make the team. None of those things are the end of the world. If I would've let fear dictate my actions, I wouldn't have done any of those things. There is a saying that goes, "To avoid criticism, do nothing, say nothing, and be nothing." And same goes for fear—if you let fear control your actions, you won't do anything that takes you out of your comfort zone, and you also won't do anything worthy in life. Sometimes doing the hard stuff makes the rest of your life seem easier because you now know what you can handle. If I would've listened to my fears, I probably wouldn't have attempted to go on my dunk journey, or gone forward with my dreams of becoming a social media influencer or a high level athlete. It doesn't get "easier" so you might still get those butterflies every time, but what happens every time you take on fear and act in spite of it, it strengthens your ability to do it again and again. Former Navy Seal, motivational speaker, ultramarathon athlete, and author of *Can't Hurt Me*, David Goggins, refers to this as "reaching into your cookie jar." The more times you accomplish something that you weren't supposed to or attempted to push harder than last time or try something new, you start adding these experiences to your cookie jar. And every time you need to find that extra gear or added motivation to try something new, you can refer to your cookie jar, reach in there and refer back to how you pushed through the challenge the last time.

And what happened with me doing the special events at camp? It started with volunteering for the little special events, then doing Simon sez and dancing. This subsequently led to doing the counselor makeover day—next I would start volunteering to go up on stage, and then I would sing/rap on stage. And as scared as I was each time, I knew that I could do it. I knew what I had been through, and this was nothing compared to what I had already overcome.

The same thing applies when you "fail" at something. There is a fear of failure or not being able to get back up again. Then, there is also the fear of success. What if I accomplish this and I can't handle it, or what if I succeed and then can't sustain it and I end up losing it all? I have experienced both types throughout my life. But, every time you realize that you get back up, and as they say get back on the bike after falling, you realize that you are okay and you can do this. You got this, and if you fail, so what—at least you have the courage to keep trying and that speaks volumes about your character. Prior to me going through my life threatening illness, if you would've told me I was gonna lose it all: my athletic abilities and all of the skills I had worked so tirelessly to achieve, the ability to jump, ability to speak, have my brain be affected, severe digestive issues, have all the health that I had focused on so intensely to buildup—have it all fall—have my whole life, my friends, the school that I had worked so hard to get into—if you would've told me I would have that all come crashing before my eyes, I wouldn't have known how to handle it. But I stuck to my principles, and I knew that I was not someone who gives up when faced with adversity. I had failed and gotten back up every other time, so I was gonna do that again. I had principles for how I lived my life, and I was on a mission no matter how long it took; I was going to live and build myself back up stronger than before. We all have this ability, and you may have to work on this. But, this is the stuff that champions are made of.

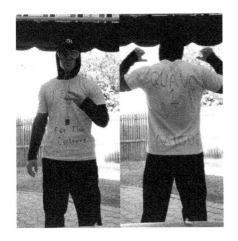
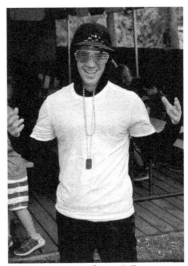

The top 2 pictures are from my performance as Quavo from Migos.

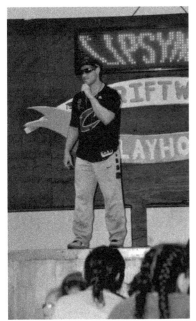
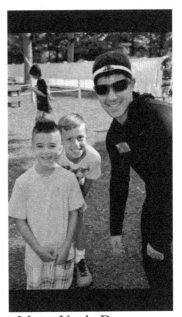

Me as Kanye Weiss.

Me as Uncle Drew.

KNOW YOUR WORTH
Chapter 80

If someone told you you were too small, too old, too young, etc., it is not a death sentence. This world doesn't know you yet! Don't give up on something if it's what you really love and what you are really passionate about. Take it as an invitation to become better than ever. It doesn't matter if you're not a star when you're 10 years old or 20 or 30 or 60; as long as you keep working at it and continue beating on your craft, you will shine when the time is right. I still haven't reached my peak in so many areas of my life. There are plenty of late bloomers out there; believe that you can be one of them, and don't quit!

If you believe in yourself and put in the necessary work to be the best, then you are worth more than a spot on the bench or just another employee of the company where you work—you need to go after what you're worth! Over the years, as I mentioned earlier, I had to deal with plenty of coaches who didn't believe in me and plenty of teammates who didn't really want me to succeed, whether it was not giving me the opportunities I felt I deserved or taking advantage of my quiet and kindhearted nature. And every time it happened, it didn't feel right or fair, and understandably so, my confidence would take a hit. The thing was, they weren't capable of seeing in me what I saw in myself. And truthfully, you shouldn't be surrounding yourself with anyone who treats you less than your best. Of course, other times in order to move up in the world or your career, you may have to play the game for a little bit. For instance, if you are working a job where you need that paycheck to support yourself/family, you may need to be careful about keeping things copacetic at work. However, this does not mean sacrificing your integrity though or ever selling out! It doesn't make it right, but there are times where in order to reach a certain spot, you may have to "play ball" for a period of time. Like for instance, how it was with my high school sports situation. As I mentioned earlier, I often wasn't given the opportunities I felt I deserved. And truthfully, I personally don't believe this was due to my skills not being up to par, and it definitely was not due to a lack of work ethic. Once again, this does not mean selling out or selling yourself short in order to please others because I would never recommend that. But sometimes part of the game is starting at the bottom, even though you know you're capable of so much more. When you first get your foot in the door, at first you may have to do basic tasks that are not exactly what you had in mind. Then, you show them what you can do and the stuff you're made of. And keep in mind, sadly, as life sometimes goes, "It's not always about what you know but who you know." But, as I also mentioned, these struggles and lack of recognition built character in me, and if I quit, I never would have actualized my full potential. Many times, however, you do need to change the situation or find a new team or new surroundings. Because unfortunately, many people will never give you the opportunity or see your full potential no matter how hard you try. Changing your environment is just as essential to success as it is to healing. As I learned, I was capable of shining under the right circumstances. But after every time I was doubted, this made me want to become so undeniably good so that I would prove these people wrong— but more importantly, prove myself right. There is no need to waste any negative energy on hating these people, but you can transform this energy into making yourself better. You do need to show some sort of forgiveness towards these people in order to become your best self, because otherwise you will carry around that negative energy.

RESULTS VS BUSYNESS
Chapter 81

I recently listened to a podcast by Andy Frisella, who happens to be one of my favorite motivational speakers and who's constantly preaching the values of hard work and not making excuses, as well as speaking some hard truths or at least what he believes to be the truth, no matter how "unpopular" it may be. However, in this particular episode he was talking about how being busy isn't an accomplishment—when we have no free time, it's a lie that we tell ourselves to make us feel like we are being more productive. In reality, efficiency and results matter, and if you're always busy maybe you have a problem with time management. So many people seemingly have this fascination with telling others how busy they are, but that doesn't mean they're actually getting stuff done. And I definitely have fallen victim to this belief as well. I used to think I had to wake up at 4:30-5 am every day to workout, and that every moment of my day had to be occupied and that I couldn't go to sleep before midnight…ever, and if I wasn't doing that, then I wasn't working hard enough. I'll say it again, "BEING BUSY IS NOT AN ACCOMPLISHMENT." And honestly that doesn't sound like too great of a life; if I have to be constantly overexerting myself and walking around like a zombie because I didn't get any sleep, then what am I working so hard for? When I realized that it's infinitely more important to get enough sleep, to maximize efficiency in my work, and to make sure I have energy for the things that matter most to me, I accomplished so much more and became so much happier. The most successful people know how to maximize their time, not just fill all of it up. My current daily routine starts with waking up after getting the amount of sleep I need. I plan my workouts and sports training based on what I feel my body needs versus just going balls to the wall 24/7. I also incorporate rest days. When I put in work on my social media posts, YouTube videos, or on this book, I make sure to take breaks and do my best to avoid distractions. I try to hang out with my inner circle as much as I can, yet still make a lot of time for alone time and meditation and self love/self care methods. At the end of every day, I write down in my journal what I hope to accomplish the next day as well as what I did during that day, trying to focus on all of the positive things that happened.

314

I find this routine to be the most effective way (for me) to get results and keep me motivated, healthy, happy, and living my best life.

I DON'T LIKE CHANGE, BUT I HAVE TO ACCEPT IT

Chapter 82

I have never been a fan of change, and especially seeing people in my life change or get older has always been tough on me. And when it comes to great times coming to an end, I always had a hard time dealing with it. Then after what I went through in 2014, my whole life just changed in the blink of an eye. I went from what I thought was a healthy college student to a kid who was fighting for my life, and I had to work so hard to get back what I had lost in the following years as well. But I also learned and gained more than I ever could have had I not gone through my healing journey. However, I think the understanding of the preciousness of each moment in life really hit me. I realized that everything could change in an instant, and I might never have that amazing experience back or see my loved ones again, and that has scared me a lot. I think this has made me hang on to things even more and attach myself to great times. I have developed some big fears, like the fear of never seeing my family and friends again. This has made me want to savor every moment I have with them and has enabled me to emotionally connect with people on a deeper level. One thing that has reduced these fears though has been my spiritual belief system and my belief that we are all eternal beings and that no matter the situation, God has a plan for me, and that plan is beyond my wildest dreams as long as I use my free will to become my highest self. I have even looked into the possibility of reincarnation; I believe our soul and our energy never actually die—therefore, I believe death isn't the end and may actually be a transformation into another realm or into our next life based on what we learned and achieved in this realm. I believe that how we choose to act in this life affects what happens next. However, there's no way of knowing 100% for sure what happens next, and that uncertainty can definitely be a bit unnerving. When people change and get older and go on about their lives, it still makes me scared and worried that they are going to leave me for good. In my amazing summers especially, I really had a tough time whenever the end would come. It would send me into a downward spiral for a few days or weeks. Even when I leave a friend's house, I sometimes get depressed that the great time is over with. Every amazing experience has a downfall when it's done. And especially with everything that I've been through, it's understandable to be afraid of going back to that "sunken place." Another fear of mine has been getting to the end of life in this current realm and current body and not having completed all of these massive goals that I set out for myself. I guess you can say this has always been the reason for my undying work ethic. It keeps me going and continuing to achieve. But I also have come to understand that it's essential to take some time to appreciate where I'm at in that moment because if we don't appreciate the moment, it will pass us by. When I started trusting God's timing, this took some of that stress away, but of course I'm human so these fears will still creep up from time to time. I really don't want things to change without my control again, but I have come to understand that some things are out of my control and I must accept that. I know what it's like to lose it all, to start from scratch and have to relearn everything. Not knowing what will come next—or if there is a next in this current form—is a very scary thought. The thought of losing everything that I've worked so hard to attain gives me a lot of anxiety. My closest friends know that I sometimes get these irrational thoughts whenever they don't text back within a day or if I don't see them for a while, because I have this deep fear that either I won't see them again, or that they don't like me, or that something happened to them. So I tell them that if I text back again, it's because I care. My obsessiveness with health and training started from a young age, and I realize I'm that way because I care. In recent years, I started getting these things called happiness hangovers. I didn't know there was a name for this at first, but after doing some research I found that I'm not alone in this. Whenever I have an amazing time with someone or if I achieve something great, I become so emotionally attached to the experience that initially my happiness hormones skyrocket, but then after a few days I realize that the experience is over and I come down into a depressed state. It's almost like when someone takes a drug—they get this huge high in emotions, and then once the drug wears off they have an equal and opposite low moment after. As I mentioned, I have never taken drugs, but the huge swing in emotions can resemble someone who does. Especially in today's society, we are constantly looking for that next hit of dopamine. In this fast paced society, we aren't taught that there's value in boredom. We go on social media, like posts, intake these quick pieces of information, crave likes and hearts, and even when we get them it's never enough. As soon as that dopamine goes away, we become sad and depressed. It's not easy being a highly sensitive person, but I think because I am so in touch with what's going on inside of me, this makes me the perfect person to understand others. I will experience the most happiness and the most sadness; that's always been my personality. Furthermore, there is a great thrill you get when you go all in on something and you display the utmost passion and enthusiasm towards it. I'm an all in or all out person, but I love myself and I wouldn't be me if I was any other way.

Practicing gratitude is super important, as well as understanding that not every moment in life can be super happy. But I also must realize that after fighting through everything that I have, I have gained incredible strength and can overcome anything. And in these more difficult moments, it's important to try to find the lesson that God wants me to learn.

With friends as well, I lay it all out there and go all in on them trying to make them feel as special as possible. Trying to make the plans work out perfectly or even just when hanging out with them, I put my all into it. This is part of who I am and I have come to accept that when you are someone who goes all out with everything, it is natural to experience the full spectrum of emotions. As Jimmy Valvano said in his famous award speech, "If you laugh, you think, and you cry, that's a full day. That's a heck of a day. You do that seven days a week, you're going to have something special."

THE BODY HAS SELF-HEALING CAPABILITIES (WHEN PLACED IN THE RIGHT ENVIRONMENT AND GIVEN THE RIGHT TOOLS FROM NATURE)

Chapter 83

One big thing that I've learned over these past 9 years is that our bodies are the most intelligent, beautiful, self healing organisms ever created. They were created perfectly by God, and they do not make mistakes. Our bodies are constantly reacting to the inputs they've been given, and this results in outputs, but ultimately they are always trying to keep us alive however they can. Sometimes this means sending us messages with pain or symptoms. Others have tried to convince us that this means our body is messing up, and it's up to the pharmaceutical industry or the government to "correct" this issue. This typically results in more illness or dis-ease, and I now understand why. We are never at war with our bodies—it's up to us to find out what our body is trying to tell us and help it with whatever it is trying to do. Getting "sick" is how our bodies rid themselves of toxins.

Doctors are often trying to label us and group us together with people based on our symptoms or our genetics or characteristics and then give us specific "medications" to treat those symptoms. But, we are constantly changing from moment to moment. You are different from anything that has ever come into this world, so you will never fit anyone's mold of you. Your whole life needs to be taken into account and needs to become your "medicine." And everyone's medicine might be different, but every moment with every input we give our bodies, we are either giving our bodies harmful inputs, whether they be spiritual, chemical, physical, interpersonal, etc., or we are providing our bodies with just what they need to allow them to do their jobs of healing us. *If you aren't constantly trying to level up, evolve, vibrate at a higher frequency, and become a more resilient human, then what are you doing?* This life has so much to offer us, but it's up to us to take it in and to realize how special we are. Out of all the people who could have entered this universe, we were chosen, and I believe we also chose to be here at this time. Some people don't want you to realize how special and how powerful you can become because then you won't need them. But you can heal from anything, overcome anything, and achieve anything. As Daniel Larusso says in Cobra Kai, "You're the only one who can get up when you're down. No one else." So you have to be the one to put the work in. Others can guide you and help you find the right path, as Victor and Cassie have done for me, but then it's up to you to do what it takes and to do what resonates with you. There is no magic pill that will heal you instantly or make it so you don't have to put up with any challenges or discomfort. There are no shortcuts, but I believe the body can heal when placed in the right environment and when given the right tools.

As Victor recently wrote about, it's never the label or diagnosis that heals you, yet we are so keen on searching for our diagnosis. Meanwhile, so many misdiagnoses happen every year. And these often carry a lot of weight with them. As many of the people I follow often talk about, it's important to shed these labels as a way of not allowing your mind to identify with that sickened state. It takes time, effort, and making sure your inputs are promoting health rather than keeping you in this state of dis-ease. But it can be done.

As Victor often says, he doesn't manage disease, he promotes wellness. We've been taught that each disease is its own specific entity caused by a different set of microscopic particles, but as I've learned, this is not the case. You don't heal or prevent disease by attacking the healing responses in the body. You promote overall wellness: help the body by placing it in the right environment, remove whatever doesn't contribute to wellness, help the body detoxify and offload all the toxins, as well as shield the body from non-native frequencies whenever possible—and most importantly connect with nature and connect with what you love and what feels right to you.

BORN READY, BUT BUILT LEGENDARY
Chapter 84

You're probably wondering, "Whatever happened with his dunk journey? Did he ever get there? He didn't finish telling that part of the story." So, here it is. Success isn't a straight path, and there's no such thing as can't; often you just have to find another way. When I was in 9th grade, the only time I ever had my vertical jump tested in high school, I tested at 23 inches standing, and it wasn't much higher running. Throughout high school, due to being severely overtrained, overstressed, sleep deprived, and often injured—my vertical by the end of high school was probably around 25-26 inches (possibly a bit higher), if I had to guess. If you remember, I had calculated that I would need a 36 inch jump to touch the rim and a few inches more to dunk. As you read about, post-hospital during the years while I was going through my healing process and starting from ground zero, I slowly began progressing. By the end of 2015, I was at 32 inches running. Then, those pesky ankle injuries derailed me a bit. I built back up, and by the end of 2016 I was at 35 inches, just one inch away from the rim. Then, the back, elbow, more ankle, and shoulder injuries came along, and for the next two years I was stuck and couldn't really jump without pain. With the help of Bodmechanic, I was able to get my muscles and bones all healed enough to jump without pain. Then, by the end of 2017, I was back up to around a 32 inch jump. But, by then my health issues were full blown, and as you know I couldn't digest foods, and the neurological issues were incredibly debilitating as my body was in a state of disrepair. All of 2018 was spent searching to find the solution to my health problems. In 2019, while I had begun following the first naturopath's program, although I still was battling through a ton, I managed to reach 36 inches and touched the rim! Over the next year, I continued fighting through significant challenges and was still far from better yet. My inconsistent energy and sleep schedule as well as all of my other health issues made it difficult to improve, but I was not going to stop trying. By the end of 2020 and into 2021 as you guys read about, I experienced the first glimpse of hope as I slowly began to navigate my way out of my health problems with my new knowledge of holistic health and incredible guidance. Although, I had to be incredibly patient and give the holistic healing time to work because as I've mentioned, healing is often uncomfortable, not easy, and not pretty. And the detoxing that has ultimately helped me so much, can also make you feel more tired and worse at times before you get better. My running vertical was stuck at around 33 inches for most of the summer of 2021. At the start of summer 2022, I was at a 27.5 inch standing jump and 33 inch running jump. As the summer progressed onward, I hit 33.5 inches and 28 inches standing, then reached 34.5 inches by the end of that summer. The summer of 2023, I was able to reach my all time standing jump PR of 29 inches and still finished at around 34.5 inches running. Then in the recent months of 2024, as you can see from the cover of the book, I am jumping my highest ever and have likely reached past 36 inches on my running jump as I am now touching the top of the rim! With my dedication to training, understanding my body better when it comes to my healing and detoxing journey—and a refusal to give up, I was able to accomplish this. I have also hit all of my highest weights lifted this past year as well, which I recorded in the epilogue... and I will continue to keep at it and will continue to improve! As motivational speaker Les Brown famously said, "IT'S NOT OVER UNTIL I WIN!"

Much of the time in life, things don't happen exactly WHEN we want them to or when we think they should. We may think that something has to happen by a certain date, or if not, then it's time to give up. That couldn't be farther from the truth. I firmly believe that God was, and is, always working on my storybook ending—it is just up to me to see it through to completion! I have to trust His timing and understand that every struggle is meant to teach me something new. So now my final words of this book: Go out there and shed your labels, shed your prior beliefs as to what's possible, and write your own story!

EPILOGUE AND ADDITIONAL THOUGHTS

My current dietary principles I follow:

Today, after tons of research during my health issues and through life experience, I discovered that it's not as much about being on a "name diet" or avoiding any specific foods as it is about preparing the foods the right way and getting them from the correct sources, as well as following what makes YOU feel and perform at your best. The food preparation and sourcing of the foods considerably alter the nutrition aspects and digestibility. It's not simply about "you are what you eat," and it's definitely so much more than just "calories in calories out," but rather you are what you can absorb and digest. Also, your mental state while you're eating matters a lot as well. If you have a good relationship with food and are happy while you eat it, and you make it into a great experience, whether with music or a podcast, or use it as a fun way to incorporate family and friends, this will translate into better health! It's also important to minimize toxins from food as much as possible by going organic. This encompasses obtaining food from high quality farms when you can (such as Miller's Bio Farm-one of my favorites), avoiding processed unnatural foods, as well as preparing the majority of your own food as this will play a role in your healing process. Many of the current diet principles I follow come from the Weston A. Price Foundation who promotes ancestral based nutrition. Also, as any of my followers or Lifetime gym people know, you will never see me without a coconut water, which I believe is one of the keys to life, as well as probably the most hydrating drink on Earth! And by being the change and modeling it for others, I have even inspired many others to start drinking it as well!

*Some of my current quantifiable numbers from today and accomplishments are as follows (keep in mind these have all been within the past few years while on my healing journey): PR for made free throws in a row with 80 and went 99/100, my PR for NBA 3 pointers in a row with 22, PR for juggling a soccer ball with over 220, and my jumping you saw in the final chapter...

Weightlifting and running numbers: Power Clean-230 lbs
Back Squat-345 lbs Bench Press-250 lbs (also 225x4 205x7) Power
Snatch-160 lbs Conventional Deadlift-375 lbs Trap Bar Deadlift: Probably
over 400 lbs. Also, a huge part of my training has become sprint training.
There is something that I absolutely love about going all out on a run and
trying to beat my time by tenths of a second. My times have improved
greatly as I keep trying to become a freakier athlete. And even through my
health struggles, my dad and I would go to the track. I brought my
unofficial 40 yard dash time from around a 5.10 to a 4.62, and my speed
on the "sprint"/curved treadmill at my gym is up to 16.7 mph top speed
as I continue to get stronger and faster. I love sprinting and it translates
well into all athletic activities. Thankfully, this also fits my build today at
5'6 170-180 lbs.
(All of these numbers increased post high school and post college, and in
my case while healing from significant health issues, so remember that
where you are today doesn't have to be where you are 5 years from now).
AND ALL THESE NUMBERS ARE STILL GOING UP AND WILL
LIKELY BE EVEN HIGHER BY THE TIME YOU READ THIS
BOOK...

My original plan was for this book to be released when both my
healing journey was "complete" and I got my first dunk on 10
feet... (Although as I've learned, the body is always healing, and
healing is in fact a journey not a destination.) However, what I've
come to realize, as you read about...things don't have to be perfect
for your story to matter, and if you wait for the perfect time, it may
never come or you might miss your chance! I know how powerful
my story and all the lessons gained along the way are right now, and
I am "perfectly imperfect..." in other words, I am right where I am
meant to be on my journeys. I know that what is meant for me will
come my way! And there is a good chance that by the time you read
this book or shortly after, those MASSIVE GOALS of mine will
have been accomplished, and if not, just know that I am working
on them! Follow along on all my social media to stay up to date.

YouTube: Jared and James
2nd YouTube for truther content: Rabbit Hole Roundup
Spotify, Apple Podcast, any audio platform: Jared and James
IG: @jaredweiss817 and truther IG: @jared_weiss
Facebook: Jared Weiss
TikTok: @jaredweiss817 and @rabbitholeroundup
Rumble: JaredandJames
Twitter/X: @jaredweiss817

And speaking of which, one last thing, I wanted to give a special thank you to all of my podcast guests who have come on and those who will come on in the future! There were so many incredible podcasts filmed just prior to releasing this book, and I wish I could give you all a shoutout, but just know how much it means to me! And furthermore, for any and all of my supporters whether it be on social media or on any of my journeys, just know how much that support means to me!

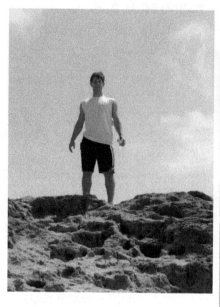

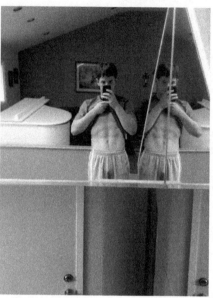

BEFORE THE ILLNESS…

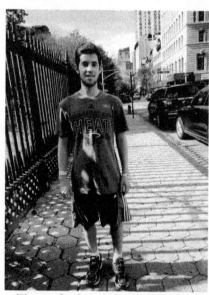

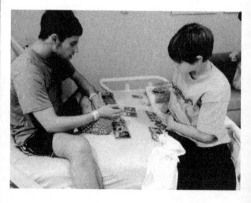

Towards the end of my hospital stay…

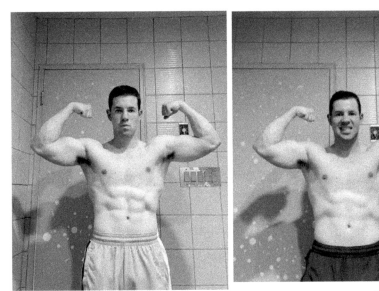

Currently…better than ever and stronger physically, mentally, and spiritually—and only getting better with time!

Fight Through It